D1721970

I. GLOSSARY

INTRODUCTION

Good Clinical Practice (GCP) is an international ethical and scientific quality standard for designing, conducting, recording and reporting trials that involve the participation of human subjects. Compliance with this standard provides public assurance that the rights, safety and well-being of trial subjects are protected, consistent with the principles that have their origin in the Declaration of Helsinki, and that the clinical trial data are credible.

The objective of this ICH GCP Guideline is to provide a unified standard for the European Union (EU), Japan and the United States to facilitate the mutual acceptance of clinical data by the regulatory authorities in these jurisdictions.

The guideline was developed with consideration of the current good clinical practices of the European Union, Japan, and the United States, as well as those of Australia, Canada, the Nordic countries and the World Health Organization (WHO).

This guideline should be followed when generating clinical trial data that are intended to be submitted to regulatory authorities.

The principles established in this guideline may also be applied to other clinical investigations that may have an impact on the safety and well-being of human subjects.

1.1 Adverse Drug Reaction (ADR)

In the pre-approval clinical experience with a new medicinal product or its new usages, particularly as the therapeutic dose(s) may not be established: all noxious and unintended responses to a medicinal product related to any dose should be considered adverse drug reactions. The phrase responses to a medicinal product means that a causal relationship between a medicinal product and an adverse event is at least a reasonable possibility, ie. the relationship cannot be ruled out.

Regarding marketed medicinal products: a response to a drug which is noxious and unintended and which occurs at doses normally used in man for prophylaxis, diagnosis, or therapy of diseases or for modification of physiological function (see the ICH Guideline for Clinical Safety Data Management: Definitions and Standards for Expedited Reporting).

1.2 Adverse Event (AE)

Any untoward medical occurrence in a patient or clinical investigation subject administered a pharmaceutical product and which does not necessarily have a causal relationship with this treatment. An adverse event (AE) can therefore be any unfavourable and unintended sign (including an abnormal laboratory finding), symptom, or disease temporally associated with the use of a medicinal (investigational) product, whether or not related to the medicinal (investigational) product (see the ICH Guideline for Clinical Safety Data Management: Definitions and Standards for Expedited Reporting).

1.3 Amendment (to the protocol)

See Protocol Amendment.

1.4 Applicable Regulatory Requirement(s)

Any law(s) and regulation(s) addressing the conduct of clinical trials of investigational products.

1.5 Approval (in relation to Institutional Review Boards)

The affirmative decision of the IRB that the clinical trial has been reviewed and may be conducted at the institution site within the constraints set forth by the IRB, the institution, Good Clinical Practice (GCP), and the applicable regulatory requirements.

1.6 Audit

A systematic and independent examination of trial related activities and documents to determine whether the evaluated trial related activities were conducted, and the data were recorded, analyzed and accurately reported according to the protocol, sponsor's standard operating procedures (SOPs), Good Clinical Practice (GCP), and the applicable regulatory requirement(s).

1.7 Audit Certificate

A declaration of confirmation by the auditor that an audit has taken place.

1.8 Audit Report

A written evaluation by the sponsor's auditor of the results of the audit.

1.9 Audit Trail

Documentation that allows reconstruction of the course of events.

1.10 Blinding/Masking

A procedure in which one or more parties to the trial are kept unaware of the treatment assignment(s). Single-blinding usually refers to the subject(s) being unaware, and double-blinding usually refers to the subject(s), investigator(s), monitor, and, in some cases, data analyst(s) being unaware of the treatment assignment(s).

1.11 Case Report Form (CRF)

A printed, optical, or electronic document designed to record all of the protocol required information to be reported to the sponsor on each trial subject.

1.12 Clinical Trial/Study

Any investigation in human subjects intended to discover or verify the clinical, pharmacological and/or other pharmacodynamic effects of an investigational product(s), and/or to identify any adverse reactions to an investigational product(s), and/or to study absorption, distribution, metabolism, and excretion of an investigational product(s) with the object of ascertaining its safety and/or efficacy. The terms clinical trial and clinical study are synonymous.

1.13 Clinical Trial/Study Report

A written description of a trial/study of any therapeutic, prophylactic, or diagnostic agent conducted in human subjects, in which the clinical and statistical description, presentations, and analyses are fully integrated into a single report (see the ICH Guideline for Structure and Content of Clinical Study Reports).

1.14 Comparator (Product)

An investigational or marketed product (ie. active control), or placebo, used as a reference in a clinical trial.

1.15 Compliance (in relation to trials)

Adherence to all the trial-related requirements, Good Clinical Practice (GCP) requirements, and the applicable regulatory requirements.

1.16 Confidentiality

Prevention of disclosure, to other than authorized individuals, of a sponsor's proprietary information or of a subject's identity.

1.17 Contract

A written, dated, and signed agreement between two or more involved parties that sets out any arrangements on delegation and distribution of tasks and obligations and, if appropriate, on financial matters. The protocol may serve as the basis of a contract.

1.18 Coordinating Committee

A committee that a sponsor may organize to coordinate the conduct of a multicentre trial.

1.19 Coordinating Investigator

An investigator assigned the responsibility for the coordination of investigators at different centres participating in a multicentre trial.

1.20 Contract Research Organization (CRO)

A person or an organization (commercial, academic, or other) contracted by the sponsor to perform one or more of a sponsor's trial-related duties and functions.

1.21 Direct Access

Permission to examine, analyze, verify, and reproduce any records and reports that are important to evaluation of a clinical trial. Any party (e.g., domestic and foreign regulatory authorities, sponsor's monitors and auditors) with direct access should take all reasonable precautions within the constraints of the applicable regulatory requirement(s) to maintain the confidentiality of subjects' identities and sponsor's proprietary information.

1.22 Documentation

All records, in any form (including, but not limited to, written, electronic, magnetic, and optical records, and scans, x-rays, and electrocardiograms) that describe or record the methods, conduct, and/or results of a trial, the factors affecting a trial, and the actions taken.

1.23 Essential Documents

Documents which individually and collectively permit evaluation of the conduct of a study and the quality of the data produced (see 8. Essential Documents for the Conduct of a Clinical Trial).

1.24 Good Clinical Practice (GCP)

A standard for the design, conduct, performance, monitoring, auditing, recording, analyses, and reporting of clinical trials that provides assurance that the data and reported results are credible and accurate, and that the rights, integrity, and confidentiality of trial subjects are protected.

1.25 Independent Data-Monitoring Committee (IDMC) (Data and Safety Monitoring Board, Monitoring Committee, Data Monitoring Committee)

An independent data-monitoring committee that may be established by the sponsor to assess at intervals the progress of a clinical trial, the safety data, and the critical efficacy endpoints, and to recommend to the sponsor whether to continue, modify, or stop a trial.

1.26 Impartial Witness

A person, who is independent of the trial, who cannot be unfairly influenced by people involved with the trial, who attends the informed consent process if the subject or the subject's legally acceptable representative cannot read, and who reads the informed consent form and any other written information supplied to the subject.

1.27 Independent Ethics Committee (IEC)

An independent body (a review board or a committee, institutional, regional, national, or supranational), constituted of medical/scientific professionals and non-medical/non-scientific members, whose responsibility it is to ensure the protection of the rights, safety and well-being of human subjects involved in a trial and to provide public assurance of that protection, by, among other things, reviewing and approving/providing favourable opinion on, the trial protocol, the suitability of the investigator(s), facilities, and the methods and material to be used in obtaining and documenting informed consent of the trial subjects.

The legal status, composition, function, operations and regulatory requirements pertaining to Independent Ethics Committees may differ among countries, but should allow the Independent Ethics Committee to act in agreement with GCP as described in this guideline.

1.28 Informed Consent

A process by which a subject voluntarily confirms his or her willingness to participate in a particular trial, after having been informed of all aspects of the trial that are relevant to the subject's decision to participate. Informed consent is documented by means of a written, signed and dated informed consent form.

1.29 Inspection

The act by a regulatory authority(ies) of conducting an official review of documents, facilities, records, and any other resources that are deemed by the authority(ies) to be related to the clinical trial and that may be located at the site of the trial, at the sponsor's and/or contract research organization's (CRO's) facilities, or at other establishments deemed appropriate by the regulatory authority(ies).

1.30 Institution (medical)

Any public or private entity or agency or medical or dental facility where clinical trials are conducted.

1.31 Institutional Review Board (IRB)

An independent body constituted of medical, scientific, and non-scientific members, whose responsibility is to ensure the protection of the rights, safety and well-being of human subjects involved in a trial by, among other things, reviewing, approving, and providing continuing review of trial protocol and amendments and of the methods and material to be used in obtaining and documenting informed consent of the trial subjects.

1.32 Interim Clinical Trial/ Study Report

A report of intermediate results and their evaluation based on analyses performed during the course of a trial.

1.33 Investigational Product

A pharmaceutical form of an active ingredient or placebo being tested or used as a reference in a clinical trial, including a product with a marketing authorization when used or assembled (formulated or packaged) in a way different from the approved form, or when used for an unapproved indication, or when used to gain further information about an approved use.

1.34 Investigator

A person responsible for the conduct of the clinical trial at a trial site. If a trial is conducted by a team of individuals at a trial site, the investigator is the responsible leader of the team and may be called the principal investigator. See also *Subinvestigator*.

1.35 Investigator / Institution

An expression meaning "the investigator and/or institution, where required by the applicable regulatory requirements".

1.36 Investigator's Brochure

A compilation of the clinical and nonclinical data on the investigational product(s) which is relevant to the study of the investigational product(s) in human subjects (see *7. Investigator's Brochure*).

1.37 Legally Acceptable Representative

An individual or juridical or other body authorized under applicable law to consent, on behalf of a prospective subject, to the subject's participation in the clinical trial.

1.38 Monitoring

The act of overseeing the progress of a clinical trial, and of ensuring that it is conducted, recorded, and reported in accordance with the protocol, Standard Operating Procedures (SOPs), Good Clinical Practice (GCP), and the applicable regulatory requirement(s).

1.39 Monitoring Report

A written report from the monitor to the sponsor after each site visit and/or other trial-related communication according to the sponsor's SOPs.

1.40 Multicentre Trial

A clinical trial conducted according to a single protocol but at more than one site, and, therefore, carried out by more than one investigator.

1.41 Nonclinical Study

Biomedical studies not performed on human subjects.

1.42 Opinion (in relation to Independent Ethics Committee)

The judgement and/or the advice provided by an Independent Ethics Committee (IEC).

1.43 Original Medical Record

See Source Documents.

1.44 Protocol

A document that describes the objective(s), design, methodology, statistical considerations, and organization of a trial. The protocol usually also gives the background and rationale for the trial, but these could be provided in other protocol referenced documents. Throughout the ICH GCP Guideline the term protocol refers to protocol and protocol amendments.

1.45 Protocol Amendment

A written description of a change(s) to or formal clarification of a protocol.

1.46 Quality Assurance (QA)

All those planned and systematic actions that are established to ensure that the trial is performed and the data are generated, documented (recorded), and reported in compliance with Good Clinical Practice (GCP) and the applicable regulatory requirement(s).

1.47 Quality Control (QC)

The operational techniques and activities undertaken within the quality assurance system to verify that the requirements for quality of the trial-related activities have been fulfilled.

1.48 Randomization

The process of assigning trial subjects to treatment or control groups using an element of chance to determine the assignments in order to reduce bias.

1.49 Regulatory Authorities

Bodies having the power to regulate. In the ICH GCP guideline the expression Regulatory Authorities includes the authorities that review submitted clinical data and those that conduct inspections (see 1.29). These bodies are sometimes referred to as competent authorities.

1.50 Serious Adverse Event (SAE) or Serious Adverse Drug Reaction (Serious ADR)

Any untoward medical occurrence that at any dose:

- results in death,
- is life-threatening,
- requires inpatient hospitalization or prolongation of existing hospitalization,
- results in persistent or significant disability/incapacity,

or

- is a congenital anomaly/birth defect (see the ICH Guideline for Clinical Safety Data Management: Definitions and Standards for Expedited Reporting).

1.51 Source Data

All information in original records and certified copies of original records of clinical findings, observations, or other activities in a clinical trial necessary for the reconstruction and evaluation of the trial. Source data are contained in source documents (original records or certified copies).

1.52 Source Documents

Original documents, data, and records (eg. hospital records, clinical and office charts, laboratory notes, memoranda, subjects' diaries or evaluation checklists, pharmacy dispensing records, recorded data from automated instruments,copies or transcriptions certified after verification as being accurate copies, microfiches, photographic negatives, microfilm or magnetic media, x-rays, subject files, and records kept at the pharmacy, at the laboratories and at medico-technical departments involved in the clinical trial).

1.53 Sponsor

An individual, company, institution, or organization which takes responsibility for the initiation, management, and/or financing of a clinical trial.

1.54 Sponsor-Investigator

An individual who both initiates and conducts, alone or with others, a clinical trial, and under whose immediate direction the investigational product is administered to, dispensed to, or used by a subject. The term does not include any person other than an individual (eg. it does not include a corporation or an agency). The obligations of a sponsor-investigator include both those of a sponsor and those of an investigator.

1.55 Standard Operating Procedures (SOPs)

Detailed, written instructions to achieve uniformity of the performance of a specific function.

1.56 Subinvestigator

Any individual member of the clinical trial team designated and supervised by the investigator at a trial site to perform critical trial-related procedures and/or to make important trial-related decisions (eg. associates, residents, research fellows). See also *Investigator*.

1.57 Subject/Trial Subject

An individual who participates in a clinical trial, either as a recipient of the investigational product(s) or as a control.

1.58 Subject Identification Code

A unique identifier assigned by the investigator to each trial subject to protect the subject's identity and used in lieu of the subject's name when the investigator reports adverse events and/or other trial related data.

1.59 Trial Site

The location(s) where trial-related activities are actually conducted.

1.60 Unexpected Adverse Drug Reaction

An adverse reaction, the nature or severity of which is not consistent with the applicable product information (eg. Investigator's Brochure for an unapproved investigational product or package insert/summary of product characteristics for an approved product) (see the ICH Guideline for Clinical Safety Data Management: Definitions and Standards for Expedited Reporting).

1.61 Vulnerable Subjects

Individuals whose willingness to volunteer in a clinical trial may be unduly influenced by the expectation, whether justified or not, of benefits associated with participation, or of a retaliatory response from senior members of a hierarchy in case of refusal to participate. Examples are members of a group with a hierarchical structure, such as medical, pharmacy, dental, and nursing students, subordinate hospital and laboratory personnel, employees of the pharmaceutical industry, members of the armed forces, and persons kept in detention. Other vulnerable subjects include patients with incurable diseases, persons in nursing homes, unemployed or impoverished persons, patients in emergency situations, ethnic minority groups, homeless persons, nomads, refugees, minors, and those incapable of giving consent.

1.62 Well-being (of the trial subjects)

The physical and mental integrity of the subjects participating in a clinical trial.

2. THE PRINCIPLES OF ICH GCP

2.1 Clinical trials should be conducted in accordance with the ethical principles that have their origin in the Declaration of Helsinki, and that are consistent with GCP and the applicable regulatory requirement(s).

2.2 Before a trial is initiated, foreseeable risks and inconveniences should be weighed against the anticipated benefit for the individual trial subject and society. A trial should be initiated and continued only if the anticipated benefits justify the risks.

2.3 The rights, safety, and well-being of the trial subjects are the most important considerations and should prevail over interests of science and society.

2.4 The available nonclinical and clinical information on an investigational product should be adequate to support the proposed clinical trial.

2.5 Clinical trials should be scientifically sound, and described in a clear, detailed protocol.

2.6 A trial should be conducted in compliance with the protocol that has received prior institutional review board (IRB)/independent ethics committee (IEC) approval/favourable opinion.

2.7 The medical care given to, and medical decisions made on behalf of, subjects should always be the responsibility of a qualified physician or, when appropriate, of a qualified dentist.

2.8 Each individual involved in conducting a trial should be qualified by education, training, and experience to perform his or her respective task(s).

2.9 Freely given informed consent should be obtained from every subject prior to clinical trial participation.

2.10 All clinical trial information should be recorded, handled, and stored in a way that allows its accurate reporting, interpretation and verification.

2.11 The confidentiality of records that could identify subjects should be protected, respecting the privacy and confidentiality rules in accordance with the applicable regulatory requirement(s).

2.12 Investigational products should be manufactured, handled, and stored in accordance with applicable good manufacturing practice (GMP). They should be used in accordance with the approved protocol.

2.13 Systems with procedures that assure the quality of every aspect of the trial should be implemented.

3. INSTITUTIONAL REVIEW BOARD/ INDEPENDENT ETHICS COMMITTEE (IRB/IEC)

3.1 Responsibilities

3.1.1 An IRB/IEC should safeguard the rights, safety, and well-being of all trial subjects. Special attention should be paid to trials that may include vulnerable subjects.

3.1.2 The IRB/IEC should obtain the following documents: trial protocol(s)/amendment(s), written informed consent form(s) and consent form updates that the investigator proposes for use in the trial, subject recruitment procedures (eg. advertisements), written information to be provided to subjects, Investigator's Brochure (IB), available safety information, information about payments and compensation available to subjects, the investigator's current curriculum vitae and/or other documentation evidencing qualifications, and any other documents that the IRB/IEC may need to fulfil its responsibilities.

The IRB/IEC should review a proposed clinical trial within a reasonable time and document its views in writing, clearly identifying the trial, the documents reviewed and the dates for the following:

– approval/favourable opinion;

– modifications required prior to its approval/favourable opinion;

– disapproval/negative opinion; and

– termination/suspension of any prior approval/favourable opinion.

3.1.3 The IRB/IEC should consider the qualifications of the investigator for the proposed trial, as documented by a current curriculum vitae and/or by any other relevant documentation the IRB/IEC requests.

3.1.4 The IRB/IEC should conduct continuing review of each ongoing trial at intervals appropriate to the degree of risk to human subjects, but at least once per year.

3.1.5 The IRB/IEC may request more information than is outlined in paragraph 4.8.10 be given to subjects when, in the judgement of the IRB/IEC, the additional information would add meaningfully to the protection of the rights, safety and/or well-being of the subjects.

3.1.6 When a non-therapeutic trial is to be carried out with the consent of the subject's legally acceptable representative (see 4.8.12, 4.8.14), the IRB/IEC should determine that

11

the proposed protocol and/or other document(s) adequately addresses relevant ethical concerns and meets applicable regulatory requirements for such trials.

3.1.7 Where the protocol indicates that prior consent of the trial subject or the subject's legally acceptable representative is not possible (see 4.8.15), the IRB/IEC should determine that the proposed protocol and/or other document(s) adquately addresses relevant ethical concerns and meets applicable regulatory requirements for such trials (ie. in emergency situations).

3.1.8 The IRB/IEC should review both the amount and method of payment to subjects to assure that neither presents problems of coercion or undue influence on the trial subjects. Payments to a subject should be prorated and not wholly contingent on completion of the trial by the subject.

3.1.9 The IRB/IEC should ensure that information regarding payment to subjects, including the methods, amounts, and schedule of payment to trial subjects, is set forth in the written informed consent form and any other written information to be provided to subjects. The way payment will be prorated should be specified.

3.2 Composition, Functions and Operations

3.2.1 The IRB/IEC should consist of a reasonable number of members, who collectively have the qualifications and experience to review and evaluate the science, medical aspects, and ethics of the proposed trial. It is recommended that the IRB/IEC should include:

(a) At least five members.

(b) At least one member whose primary area of interest is in a non-scientific area.

(c) At least one member who is independent of the institution/trial site.

Only those IRB/IEC members who are independent of the investigator and the sponsor of the trial should vote/provide opinion on a trial-related matter.

A list of IRB/IEC members and their qualifications should be maintained.

3.2.2 The IRB/IEC should perform its functions according to written operating procedures, should maintain written records of its activities and minutes of its meetings, and should comply with GCP and with the applicable regulatory requirement(s).

3.2.3 An IRB/IEC should make its decisions at announced meetings at which at least a quorum, as stipulated in its written operating procedures, is present.

3.2.4 Only members who participate in the IRB/IEC review and discussion should vote/provide their opinion and/or advise.

3.2.5 The investigator may provide information on any aspect of the trial, but should not participate in the deliberations of the IRB/IEC or in the vote/opinion of the IRB/IEC.

3.2.6 An IRB/IEC may invite non-members with expertise in special areas for assistance.

3.3 Procedures

The IRB/IEC should establish, document in writing, and follow its procedures, which should include:

3.3.1 Determining its composition (names and qualifications of the members) and the authority under which it is established.

3.3.2 Scheduling, notifying its members of, and conducting its meetings.

3.3.3 Conducting initial and continuing review of trials.

3.3.4 Determining the frequency of continuing review, as appropriate.

3.3.5 Providing, according to the applicable regulatory requirements, expedited review and approval/favourable opinion of minor change(s) in ongoing trials that have the approval/ favourable opinion of the IRB/IEC.

3.3.6 Specifying that no subject should be admitted to a trial before the IRB/IEC issues its written approval/ favourable opinion of the trial.

3.3.7 Specifying that no deviations from, or changes of, the protocol should be initiated without prior written IRB/IEC approval/favourable opinion of an appropriate amendment, except when necessary to eliminate immediate hazards to the subjects or when the change(s) involves only logistical or administrative aspects of the trial (eg. change of monitor(s), telephone number(s)) (see 4.5.2).

3.3.8 Specifying that the investigator should promptly report to the IRB/IEC:

(a) Deviations from, or changes of, the protocol to eliminate immediate hazards to the trial subjects (see 3.3.7, 4.5.2, 4.5.4).
(b) Changes increasing the risk to subjects and/or affecting significantly the conduct of the trial (see 4.10.2).
(c) All adverse drug reactions (ADRs) that are both serious and unexpected.
(d) New information that may affect adversely the safety of the subjects or the conduct of the trial.

3.3.9 Ensuring that the IRB/IEC promptly notify in writing the investigator/institution concerning:

(a) Its trial-related decisions/opin-
ions.
(b) The reasons for its decisions/
opinions.
(c) Procedures for appeal of its
decisions/opinions.

3.4 Records
The IRB/IEC should retain all relevant records (eg. written procedures, membership lists, lists of
occupations/affiliations of members,
submitted documents, minutes of
meetings, and correspondence) for a
period of at least 3 years after completion of the trial and make them
available upon request from the regulatory authority(ies).

The IRB/IEC may be asked by investigators, sponsors or regulatory
authorities to provide its written
procedures and membership lists.

4. INVESTIGATOR

4.1 Investigator's Qualifications and Agreements

4.1.1 The investigator(s) should be qualified by education, training, and experience to assume responsibility for the proper conduct of the trial, should meet all the qualifications specified by the applicable regulatory requirement(s), and should provide evidence of such qualifications through up-to-date curriculum vitae and/or other relevant documentation requested by the sponsor, the IRB/IEC, and/or the regulatory authority(ies).

4.1.2 The investigator should be thoroughly familiar with the appropriate use of the investigational product(s), as described in the protocol, in the current Investigator's Brochure, in the product information and in other information sources provided by the sponsor.

4.1.3 The investigator should be aware of, and should comply with, GCP and the applicable regulatory requirements.

4.1.4 The investigator/institution should permit monitoring and auditing by the sponsor, and inspection by the appropriate regulatory authority(ies).

4.1.5 The investigator should maintain a list of appropriately qualified persons to whom the investigator has delegated significant trial-related duties.

4.2 Adequate Resources

4.2.1 The investigator should be able to demonstrate (eg. based on retrospective data) a potential for recruiting the required number of suitable subjects within the agreed recruitment period.

4.2.2 The investigator should have sufficient time to properly conduct and complete the trial within the agreed trial period.

4.2.3 The investigator should have available an adequate number of qualified staff and adequate facilities for the foreseen duration of the trial to conduct the trial properly and safely.

4.2.4 The investigator should ensure that all persons assisting with the trial are adequately informed about the protocol, the investigational product(s), and their trial-related duties and functions.

4.3 Medical Care of Trial Subjects

4.3.1 A qualified physician (or dentist, when appropriate), who is an investigator or a sub-investigator for the trial, should be responsible for all trial-related medical (or dental) decisions.

4.3.2 During and following a subject's participation in a trial, the investigator/institution should ensure that adequate medical care is provided to a subject for any adverse events, including clinically significant laboratory values, related to the trial. The investigator/institution should inform a subject when medical care is needed for intercurrent illness(es) of which the investigator becomes aware.

4.3.3 It is recommended that the investigator inform the subject's primary physician about the subject's participation in the trial if the subject has a primary physician and if the subject agrees to the primary physician being informed.

4.3.4 Although a subject is not obliged to give his/her reason(s) for withdrawing prematurely from a trial, the investigator should make a reasonable effort to ascertain the reason(s), while fully respecting the subject's rights.

4.4 Communication with IRB/IEC

4.4.1 Before initiating a trial, the investigator/institution should have written and dated approval/favourable opinion from the IRB/IEC for the trial protocol, written

informed consent form, consent form updates, subject recruitment procedures (eg. advertisements), and any other written information to be provided to subjects.

4.4.2 As part of the investigator's/institution's written application to the IRB/IEC, the investigator/institution should provide the IRB/IEC with a current copy of the Investigator's Brochure. If the Investigator's Brochure is updated during the trial, the investigator/institution should supply a copy of the updated Investigator's Brochure to the IRB/IEC.

4.4.3 During the trial the investigator/ institution should provide to the IRB/IEC all documents subject to review.

4.5 Compliance with Protocol

4.5.1 The investigator/institution should conduct the trial in compliance with the protocol agreed to by the sponsor and, if required, by the regulatory authority(ies) and which was given approval/favourable opinion by the IRB/IEC. The investigator/ institution and the sponsor should sign the protocol, or an alternative contract, to confirm agreement.

4.5.2 The investigator should not implement any deviation from, or changes of the protocol without agreement by the sponsor and prior review and documented approval/

favourable opinion from the IRB/IEC of an amendment, except where necessary to eliminate an immediate hazard(s) to trial subjects, or when the change(s) involves only logistical or administrative aspects of the trial (eg. change in monitor(s), change of telephone number(s)).

4.5.3 The investigator, or person designated by the investigator, should document and explain any deviation from the approved protocol.

4.5.4 The investigator may implement a deviation from, or a change of, the protocol to eliminate an immediate hazard(s) to trial subjects without prior IRB/IEC approval/ favourable opinion. As soon as possible, the implemented deviation or change, the reasons for it, and, if appropriate, the proposed protocol amendment(s) should be submitted:
(a) to the IRB/IEC for review and approval/favourable opinion,
(b) to the sponsor for agreement and, if required,
(c) to the regulatory authority(ies).

4.6 Investigational Product(s)
4.6.1 Responsibility for investigational product(s) accountability at the trial site(s) rests with the investigator/institution.

4.6.2 Where allowed/required, the investigator/institution may/should assign some or all of the investigator's/institution's duties for investigational product(s) accountability at the trial site(s) to an appropriate pharmacist or another appropriate individual who is under the supervision of the investigator/institution.

4.6.3 The investigator/institution and/or a pharmacist or other appropriate individual, who is designated by the investigator/institution, should maintain records of the product's delivery to the trial site, the inventory at the site, the use by each subject, and the return to the sponsor or alternative disposition of unused product(s). These records should include dates, quantities, batch/serial numbers, expiration dates (if applicable), and the unique code numbers assigned to the investigational product(s) and trial subjects. Investigators should maintain records that document adequately that the subjects were provided the doses specified by the protocol and reconcile all investigational product(s) received from the sponsor.

4.6.4 The investigational product(s) should be stored as specified by the sponsor (see 5.13.2 and 5.14.3) and in accordance with applicable regulatory requirement(s).

4.6.5 The investigator should ensure that the investigational product(s) are used only in accordance with the approved protocol.

4.6.6 The investigator, or a person designated by the investigator/institution, should explain the correct use of the investigational product(s) to each subject and should check, at intervals appropriate for the trial, that each subject is following the instructions properly.

4.7 Randomization Procedures and Unblinding

The investigator should follow the trial's randomization procedures, if any, and should ensure that the code is broken only in accordance with the protocol. If the trial is blinded, the investigator should promptly document and explain to the sponsor any premature unblinding (eg. accidental unblinding, unblinding due to a serious adverse event) of the investigational product(s).

4.8 Informed Consent of Trial Subjects

4.8.1 In obtaining and documenting informed consent, the investigator should comply with the applicable regulatory requirement(s), and should adhere to GCP and to the ethical principles that have their origin in the Declaration of Helsinki. Prior to the beginning of the trial, the investigator should have the IRB/IEC's written approval/favourable opinion of the written informed consent form and any other written information to be provided to subjects.

4.8.2 The written informed consent form and any other written information to be provided to subjects should be revised whenever important new information becomes available that may be relevant to the subject's consent. Any revised written informed consent form, and written information should receive the IRB/IEC's approval/favourable opinion in advance of use. The subject or the subject's legally acceptable representative should be informed in a timely manner if new information becomes available that may be relevant to the subject's willingness to continue participation in the trial. The communication of this information should be documented.

4.8.3 Neither the investigator, nor the trial staff, should coerce or unduly influence a subject to participate or to continue to participate in a trial.

4.8.4 None of the oral and written information concerning the trial, including the written informed consent form, should contain any language that causes the subject or the subject's legally acceptable representative to waive or to appear to waive any legal rights, or that releases or appears to release the investigator, the institution, the sponsor, or their agents from liability for negligence.

4.8.5 The investigator, or a person designated by the investigator, should fully inform the subject or, if the subject is unable to provide informed consent, the subject's legally acceptable representative, of all pertinent aspects of the trial including the written information given approval/favourable opinion by the IRB/IEC.

4.8.6 The language used in the oral and written information about the trial, including the written informed consent form, should be as non-technical as practical and should be understandable to the subject or the subject's legally acceptable representative and the impartial witness, where applicable.

4.8.7 Before informed consent may be obtained, the investigator, or a person designated by the investigator, should provide the subject or the subject's legally acceptable representative ample time and opportunity to inquire about details of the trial and to decide whether or not to participate in the trial. All questions about the trial should be answered to the satisfaction of the subject or the subject's legally acceptable representative.

4.8.8 Prior to a subject's participation in the trial, the written informed consent form should be signed and personally dated by the subject or by the subject's legally acceptable representative, and by the person who conducted the informed consent discussion.

4.8.9 If a subject is unable to read or if a legally acceptable representative is unable to read, an impartial witness should be present during the entire informed consent discussion. After the written informed consent form and any other written information to be provided to subjects, is read and explained to the subject or the subject's legally acceptable representative, and after the subject or the subject's legally acceptable representative has orally consented to the subject's participation in the trial and, if capable of doing so, has signed and personally dated the informed consent form, the witness should sign and personally date the consent form. By signing the consent form, the witness attests that the information in the consent form and any other written information was accurately explained to, and apparently understood by, the subject or the subject's legally acceptable representative, and that informed consent was freely given by the subject or the subject's legally acceptable representative.

4.8.10 Both the informed consent discussion and the written informed consent form and any other written information to be provided to subjects should include explanations of the following:

(a) That the trial involves research.

(b) The purpose of the trial.

(c) The trial treatment(s) and the probability for random assignment to each treatment.

(d) The trial procedures to be followed, including all invasive procedures.

(e) The subject's responsibilities.

(f) Those aspects of the trial that are experimental.

(g) The reasonably foreseeable risks or inconveniences to the subject and, when applicable, to an embryo, fetus, or nursing infant.

(h) The reasonably expected benefits. When there is no intended clinical benefit to the subject, the subject should be made aware of this.

(i) The alternative procedure(s) or course(s) of treatment that may be available to the subject, and their important potential benefits and risks.

(j) The compensation and/or treatment available to the subject in the event of trial-related injury.

(k) The anticipated prorated payment, if any, to the subject for participating in the trial.

(l) The anticipated expenses, if any, to the subject for participating in the trial.

(m) That the subject's participation in the trial is voluntary and that the subject may refuse to participate or withdraw from the trial, at any time, without penalty or loss of benefits to which the subject is otherwise entitled.

(n) That the monitor(s), the auditor(s), the IRB/IEC, and the regulatory authority(ies) will be granted direct access to the subject's original medical records for verification of clinical trial procedures and/or data, without violating the confidentiality of the subject, to the extent permitted by the applicable laws and regulations and that, by signing a written informed consent form, the subject or the subject's legally acceptable representative is authorizing such access.

(o) That records identifying the subject will be kept confidential and, to the extent permitted by the applicable laws and/or regulations, will not be made publicly available. If the results of the trial are published, the subject's identity will remain confidential.

(p) That the subject or the subject's legally acceptable representative will be informed in a timely manner if information becomes available that may be relevant to the subject's willingness to continue participation in the trial.

(q) The person(s) to contact for further information regarding the trial and the rights of trial subjects, and whom to contact in the event of trial-related injury.

(r) The foreseeable circumstances and/or reasons under which the subject's participation in the trial may be terminated.

(s) The expected duration of the subject's participation in the trial.

(t) The approximate number of subjects involved in the trial.

4.8.11 Prior to participation in the trial, the subject or the subject's legally acceptable representative should receive a copy of the signed and dated written informed consent form and any other written information provided to the subjects. During a subject's participation in the trial, the subject or the subject's legally acceptable representative should receive a copy of the signed and dated consent form updates and a copy of any amendments to the written information provided to subjects.

4.8.12 When a clinical trial (therapeutic or non-therapeutic) includes subjects who can only be enrolled in the trial with the consent of the subject's legally acceptable representative (eg. minors, or patients with severe dementia), the subject should be informed about the trial to the extent compatible with the subject's understanding and, if capable, the subject should sign and personally date the written informed consent.

4.8.13 Except as described in 4.8.14, a non-therapeutic trial (ie. a trial in which there is no anticipated direct clinical benefit to the subject), should be conducted in subjects who personally give consent and who sign and date the written informed consent form.

4.8.14 Non-therapeutic trials may be conducted in subjects with con-

sent of a legally acceptable representative provided the following conditions are fulfilled:
(a) The objectives of the trial can not be met by means of a trial in subjects who can give informed consent personally.
(b) The foreseeable risks to the subjects are low.
(c) The negative impact on the subject's well-being is minimized and low.
(d) The trial is not prohibited by law.
(e) The approval/favourable opinion of the IRB/IEC is expressly sought on the inclusion of such subjects, and the written approval/favourable opinion covers this aspect.

Such trials, unless an exception is justified, should be conducted in patients having a disease or condition for which the investigational product is intended. Subjects in these trials should be particularly closely monitored and should be withdrawn if they appear to be unduly distressed.

4.8.15 In emergency situations, when prior consent of the subject is not possible, the consent of the subject's legally acceptable representative, if present, should be requested. When prior consent of the subject is not possible, and the subject's legally acceptable representative is not available, enrolment of the subject should require measures described in the protocol and/or elsewhere, with documented approval/favourable opinion by the IRB/IEC, to protect the rights, safety and well-being of the subject and to ensure compliance with applicable regulatory requirements. The subject or the subject's legally acceptable representative should be informed about the trial as soon as possible and consent to continue and other consent as appropriate (see 4.8.10) should be requested.

4.9 Records and Reports

4.9.1 The investigator should ensure the accuracy, completeness, legibility, and timeliness of the data reported to the sponsor in the CRFs and in all required reports.

4.9.2 Data reported on the CRF, that are derived from source documents, should be consistent with the source documents or the discrepancies should be explained.

4.9.3 Any change or correction to a CRF should be dated, initialed, and explained (if necessary) and should not obscure the original entry (ie. an audit trail should be maintained); this applies to both written and electronic changes or corrections (see 5.18.4 (n)). Sponsors should provide guidance to investigators and/or the investigators' designated representatives on making such corrections. Sponsors should have written proce-

dures to assure that changes or corrections in CRFs made by sponsor's designated representatives are documented, are necessary, and are endorsed by the investigator. The investigator should retain records of the changes and corrections.

4.9.4 The investigator/institution should maintain the trial documents as specified in Essential Documents for the Conduct of a Clinical Trial (see 8.) and as required by the applicable regulatory requirement(s). The investigator/institution should take measures to prevent accidental or premature destruction of these documents.

4.9.5 Essential documents should be retained until at least 2 years after the last approval of a marketing application in an ICH region and until there are no pending or contemplated marketing applications in an ICH region or at least 2 years have elapsed since the formal discontinuation of clinical development of the investigational product. These documents should be retained for a longer period however if required by the applicable regulatory requirements or by an agreement with the sponsor. It is the responsibility of the sponsor to inform the investigator/institution as to when these documents no longer need to be retained (see 5.5.12).

4.9.6 The financial aspects of the

trial should be documented in an agreement between the sponsor and the investigator/institution.

4.9.7 Upon request of the monitor, auditor, IRB/IEC, or regulatory authority, the investigator/institution should make available for direct access all requested trial-related records.

4.10 Progress Reports
4.10.1 The investigator should submit written summaries of the trial status to the IRB/IEC annually, or more frequently, if requested by the IRB/IEC.

4.10.2 The investigator should promptly provide written reports to the sponsor, the IRB/IEC (see 3.3.8) and, where applicable, the institution on any changes significantly affecting the conduct of the trial, and/or increasing the risk to subjects.

4.11 Safety Reporting
4.11.1 All serious adverse events (SAEs) should be reported immediately to the sponsor except for those SAEs that the protocol or other document (eg. Investigator's Brochure) identifies as not needing immediate reporting. The immediate reports should be followed promptly by detailed, written reports. The immediate and follow-up reports should identify subjects by unique code numbers assigned to the trial subjects rather than by the subjects'

names, personal identification numbers, and/or addresses. The investigator should also comply with the applicable regulatory requirement(s) related to the reporting of unexpected serious adverse drug reactions to the regulatory authority(ies) and the IRB/IEC.

4.11.2 Adverse events and/or laboratory abnormalities identified in the protocol as critical to safety evaluations should be reported to the sponsor according to the reporting requirements and within the time periods specified by the sponsor in the protocol.

4.11.3 For reported deaths, the investigator should supply the sponsor and the IRB/IEC with any additional requested information (eg. autopsy reports and terminal medical reports).

4.12 Premature Termination or Suspension of a Trial
If the trial is prematurely terminated or suspended for any reason, the investigator/institution should promptly inform the trial subjects, should assure appropriate therapy and follow-up for the subjects, and, where required by the applicable regulatory requirement(s), should inform the regulatory authority(ies). In addition:

4.12.1 If the investigator terminates or suspends a trial without prior agreement of the sponsor, the investigator should inform the institution where applicable, and the investigator/institution should promptly inform the sponsor and the IRB/IEC, and should provide the sponsor and the IRB/IEC a detailed written explanation of the termination or suspension.

4.12.2 If the sponsor terminates or suspends a trial (see 5.21), the investigator should promptly inform the institution where applicable and the investigator/institution should promptly inform the IRB/IEC and provide the IRB/IEC a detailed written explanation of the termination or suspension.

4.12.3 If the IRB/IEC terminates or suspends its approval/favourable opinion of a trial (see 3.1.2 and 3.3.9), the investigator should inform the institution where applicable and the investigator/institution should promptly notify the sponsor and provide the sponsor with a detailed written explanation of the termination or suspension.

4.13 Final Report(s) by Investigator

Upon completion of the trial, the investigator, where applicable, should inform the institution; the investigator/institution should provide the IRB/IEC with a summary of the trial's outcome, and the regulatory authority(ies) with any reports required.

5. SPONSOR

5.1 Quality Assurance and Quality Control

5.1.1 The sponsor is responsible for implementing and maintaining quality assurance and quality control systems with written SOPs to ensure that trials are conducted and data are generated, documented (recorded), and reported in compliance with the protocol, GCP, and the applicable regulatory requirement(s).

5.1.2 The sponsor is responsible for securing agreement from all involved parties to ensure direct access (see 1.21) to all trial related sites, source data/documents, and reports for the purpose of monitoring and auditing by the sponsor, and inspection by domestic and foreign regulatory authorities.

5.1.3 Quality control should be applied to each stage of data handling to ensure that all data are reliable and have been processed correctly.

5.1.4 Agreements, made by the sponsor with the investigator/institution and any other parties involved with the clinical trial, should be in writing, as part of the protocol or in a separate agreement.

5.2 Contract Research Organization (CRO)

5.2.1 A sponsor may transfer any or all of the sponsor's trial-related duties and functions to a CRO, but the ultimate responsibility for the quality and integrity of the trial data always resides with the sponsor. The CRO should implement quality assurance and quality control.

5.2.2 Any trial-related duty and function that is transferred to and assumed by a CRO should be specified in writing.

5.2.3 Any trial-related duties and functions not specifically transferred to and assumed by a CRO are retained by the sponsor.

5.2.4 All references to a sponsor in this guideline also apply to a CRO to the extent that a CRO has assumed the trial related duties and functions of a sponsor.

5.3 Medical Expertise

The sponsor should designate appropriately qualified medical personnel who will be readily available to advise on trial related medical questions or problems. If necessary, outside consultant(s) may be appointed for this purpose.

5.4 Trial Design

5.4.1 The sponsor should utilize qualified individuals (eg. biostatisticians, clinical pharmacologists, and physicians) as appropriate, throughout all stages of the trial process, from designing the protocol and CRFs and planning the analyses to analyzing and preparing interim and final clinical trial reports.

5.4.2 For further guidance: Clinical Trial Protocol and Protocol Amendment(s) (see 6.), the ICH Guideline for Structure and Content of Clinical Study Reports, and other appropriate ICH guidance on trial design, protocol and conduct.

5.5 Trial Management, Data Handling, and Record Keeping

5.5.1 The sponsor should utilize appropriately qualified individuals to supervise the overall conduct of the trial, to handle the data, to verify the data, to conduct the statistical analyses, and to prepare the trial reports.

5.5.2 The sponsor may consider establishing an independent data-monitoring committee (IDMC) to assess the progress of a clinical trial, including the safety data and the critical efficacy endpoints at intervals, and to recommend to the sponsor whether to continue, modify, or stop a trial. The IDMC should have written operating procedures and maintain written records of all its meetings.

5.5.3 When using electronic trial data handling and/or remote elec-

tronic trial data systems, the sponsor should:

(a) Ensure and document that the electronic data processing system(s) conforms to the sponsor's established requirements for completeness, accuracy, reliability, and consistent intended performance (ie. validation).

(b) Maintains SOPs for using these systems.

(c) Ensure that the systems are designed to permit data changes in such a way that the data changes are documented and that there is no deletion of entered data (ie. maintain an audit trail, data trail, edit trail).

(d) Maintain a security system that prevents unauthorized access to the data.

(e) Maintain a list of the individuals who are authorized to make data changes (see 4.1.5 and 4.9.3).

(f) Maintain adequate backup of the data.

(g) Safeguard the blinding, if any (eg. maintain the blinding during data entry and processing).

5.5.4 If data are transformed during processing, it should always be possible to compare the original data and observations with the processed data.

5.5.5 The sponsor should use an unambiguous subject identification code (see 1.58) that allows identification of all the data reported for each subject.

5.5.6 The sponsor, or other owners of the data, should retain all of the sponsor-specific essential documents pertaining to the trial (see 8. Essential Documents for the Conduct of a Clinical Trial).

5.5.7 The sponsor should retain all sponsor-specific essential documents in conformance with the applicable regulatory requirement(s) of the country(ies) where the product is approved, and/or where the sponsor intends to apply for approval(s).

5.5.8 If the sponsor discontinues the clinical development of an investigational product (ie. for any or all indications, routes of administration, or dosage forms), the sponsor should maintain all sponsor-specific essential documents for at least 2 years after formal discontinuation or in conformance with the applicable regulatory requirement(s).

5.5.9 If the sponsor discontinues the clinical development of an investigational product, the sponsor should notify all the trial investigators/institutions and all the regulatory authorities.

5.5.10 Any transfer of ownership of the data should be reported to the appropriate authority(ies), as required by the applicable regulatory requirement(s).

5.5.11 The sponsor specific essential documents should be retained until at least 2 years after the last approval of a marketing application in an ICH region and until there are no pending or contemplated marketing applications in an ICH region or at least 2 years have elapsed since the formal discontinuation of clinical development of the investigational product. These documents should be retained for a longer period however if required by the applicable regulatory requirement(s) or if needed by the sponsor.

5.5.12 The sponsor should inform the investigator(s)/institution(s) in writing of the need for record retention and should notify the investigator(s)/institution(s) in writing when the trial related records are no longer needed.

5.6 Investigator Selection

5.6.1 The sponsor is responsible for selecting the investigator(s)/institution(s). Each investigator should be qualified by training and experience and should have adequate resources (see 4.1, 4.2) to properly conduct the trial for which the investigator is selected. If organization of a coordinating committee and/or selection of coordinating investigator(s) are to be utilized in multicentre trials, their organization and/or selection are the sponsor's responsibility.

5.6.2 Before entering an agreement

with an investigator/institution to conduct a trial, the sponsor should provide the investigator(s)/institution(s) with the protocol and an up-to-date Investigator's Brochure, and should provide sufficient time for the investigator/institution to review the protocol and the information provided.

5.6.3 The sponsor should obtain the investigator's/institution's agreement:

(a) to conduct the trial in compliance with GCP, with the applicable regulatory requirement(s) (see 4.1.3), and with the protocol agreed to by the sponsor and given approval/favourable opinion by the IRB/IEC (see 4.5.1);

(b) to comply with procedures for data recording/reporting;

(c) to permit monitoring, auditing and inspection (see 4.1.4) and

(d) to retain the trial related essential documents until the sponsor informs the investigator/institution these documents are no longer needed (see 4.9.4 and 5.5.12).

The sponsor and the investigator/institution should sign the protocol, or an alternative document, to confirm this agreement.

5.7 Allocation of Duties and Functions

Prior to initiating a trial, the sponsor should define, establish, and allocate all trial-related duties and functions.

5.8 Compensation to Subjects and Investigators

5.8.1 If required by the applicable regulatory requirement(s), the sponsor should provide insurance or should indemnify (legal and financial coverage) the investigator/the institution against claims arising from the trial, except for claims that arise from malpractice and/or negligence.

5.8.2 The sponsor's policies and procedures should address the costs of treatment of trial subjects in the event of trial-related injuries in accordance with the applicable regulatory requirement(s).

5.8.3 When trial subjects receive compensation, the method and manner of compensation should comply with applicable regulatory requirement(s).

5.9 Financing

The financial aspects of the trial should be documented in an agreement between the sponsor and the investigator/institution.

5.10 Notification/Submission to Regulatory Authority(ies)

Before initiating the clinical trial(s), the sponsor (or the sponsor and the investigator, if required by the applicable regulatory requirement(s)) should submit any required application(s) to the appropriate authority(ies) for review, acceptance, and/or permission (as required by the applicable regulatory require-ment(s) to begin the trial(s). Any notification/submission should be dated and contain sufficient informa-tion to identify the protocol.

5.11 Confirmation of Review by IRB/IEC

5.11.1 The sponsor should obtain from the investigator/institution:

(a) The name and address of the investigator's/institution's IRB/IEC.

(b) A statement obtained from the IRB/IEC that it is organized and operates according to GCP and the applicable laws and regula-tions.

(c) Documented IRB/IEC approval/favourable opinion and, if requested by the sponsor, a cur-rent copy of protocol, written informed consent form(s) and any other written information to be provided to subjects, subject recruiting procedures, and docu-ments related to payments and compensation available to the subjects, and any other docu-ments that the IRB/IEC may have requested.

5.11.2 If the IRB/IEC conditions its approval/favourable opinion upon change(s) in any aspect of the trial, such as modification(s) of the proto-col, written informed consent form and any other written information to be provided to subjects, and/or other procedures, the sponsor should obtain from the investigator/institution a copy of the modifica-tion(s) made and the date approval/favourable opinion was given by the IRB/IEC.

5.11.3 The sponsor should obtain from the investigator/institution doc-umentation and dates of any IRB/IEC reapprovals/re-evaluations with favourable opinion, and of any with-drawals or suspensions of approval/favourable opinion.

5.12 Information on Investigational Product(s)

5.12.1 When planning trials, the sponsor should ensure that sufficient safety and efficacy data from nonclin-ical studies and/or clinical trials are available to support human exposure by the route, at the dosages, for the duration, and in the trial population to be studied.

5.12.2 The sponsor should update the Investigator's Brochure as signifi-cant new information becomes avail-able (see 7. *Investigator's Brochure*).

5.13 Manufacturing, Packaging, Labelling, and Coding Investigational Product(s)

5.13.1 The sponsor should ensure that the investigational product(s) (including active comparator(s) and placebo, if applicable) is character-ized as appropriate to the stage of development of the product(s), is manufactured in accordance with any applicable GMP, and is coded and labelled in a manner that protects the blinding, if applicable. In addition, the labelling should comply with applicable regulatory requirement(s).

5.13.2 The sponsor should determine, for the investigational product(s), acceptable storage temperatures, storage conditions (eg. protection from light), storage times, reconstitution fluids and procedures, and devices for product infusion, if any. The sponsor should inform all involved parties (eg. monitors, investigators, pharmacists, storage managers) of these determinations.

5.13.3 The investigational product(s) should be packaged to prevent contamination and unacceptable deterioration during transport and storage.

5.13.4 In blinded trials, the coding system for the investigational product(s) should include a mechanism that permits rapid identification of the product(s) in case of a medical emergency, but does not permit undetectable breaks of the blinding.

5.13.5 If significant formulation changes are made in the investigational or comparator product(s) during the course of clinical development, the results of any additional studies of the formulated product(s) (eg. stability, dissolution rate, bioavailability) needed to assess whether these changes would significantly alter the pharmacokinetic profile of the product should be available prior to the use of the new formulation in clinical trials.

5.14 Supplying and Handling Investigational Product(s)

5.14.1 The sponsor is responsible for supplying the investigator(s)/institution(s) with the investigational product(s).

5.14.2 The sponsor should not supply an investigator/institution with the investigational product(s) until the sponsor obtains all required documentation (eg. approval/favourable opinion from IRB/IEC and regulatory authority(ies)).

5.14.3 The sponsor should ensure that written procedures include instructions that the investigator/institution should follow for the handling and storage of investigational product(s) for the trial and documentation thereof. The procedures should address adequate and safe receipt, handling, storage, dispensing, retrieval of unused product from subjects, and return of unused investigational product(s) to the sponsor (or alternative disposition if authorized by the sponsor and in compliance with the applicable regulatory requirement(s)).

5.14.4 The sponsor should:

(a) Ensure timely delivery of investigational product(s) to the investigator(s).

(b) Maintain records that document shipment, receipt, disposition, return, and destruction of the investigational product(s) (see 8. Essential Documents for the Conduct of a Clinical Trial).

(c) Maintain a system for retrieving investigational products and documenting this retrieval (eg. for deficient product recall, reclaim after trial completion, expired product reclaim).

(d) Maintain a system for the disposition of unused investigational product(s) and for the documentation of this disposition.

5.14.5 The sponsor should:

(a) Take steps to ensure that the investigational product(s) are stable over the period of use.

(b) Maintain sufficient quantities of the investigational product(s) used in the trials to reconfirm specifications, should this become necessary, and maintain records of batch sample analyses and characteristics. To the extent stability permits, samples should be retained either until the analyses of the trial data are complete or as required by the applicable regulatory requirement(s), whichever represents the longer retention period.

5.15 Record Access

5.15.1 The sponsor should ensure that it is specified in the protocol or other written agreement that the investigator(s)/institution(s) provide direct access to source data/documents for trial-related monitoring, audits, IRB/IEC review, and regulatory inspection.

5.15.2 The sponsor should verify that each subject has consented, in writing, to direct access to his/her original medical records for trial-related monitoring, audit, IRB/IEC review, and regulatory inspection.

5.16 Safety Information

5.16.1 The sponsor is responsible for the ongoing safety evaluation of the investigational product(s).

5.16.2 The sponsor should promptly notify all concerned investigator(s)/institution(s) and the regulatory authority(ies) of findings that could affect adversely the safety of subjects, impact the conduct of the trial, or alter the IRB/IEC's approval/favourable opinion to continue the trial.

5.17 Adverse Drug Reaction Reporting

5.17.1 The sponsor should expedite the reporting to all concerned investigator(s)/institutions(s), to the IRB(s)/IEC(s), where required, and to the regulatory authority(ies) of all adverse drug reactions (ADRs) that are both serious and unexpected.

5.17.2 Such expedited reports should comply with the applicable regulatory requirement(s) and with the ICH Guideline for Clinical Safety Data Management: Definitions and Standards for Expedited Reporting.

5.17.3 The sponsor should submit to the regulatory authority(ies) all safety updates and periodic reports, as required by applicable regulatory requirement(s).

5.18 Monitoring

5.18.1 *Purpose*

The purposes of trial monitoring are to verify that:

(a) The rights and well-being of human subjects are protected.

(b) The reported trial data are accurate, complete, and verifiable from source documents.

(c) The conduct of the trial is in compliance with the currently approved protocol/amendment(s), with GCP, and with the applicable regulatory requirement(s).

5.18.2 *Selection and Qualifications of Monitors*

(a) Monitors should be appointed by the sponsor.

(b) Monitors should be appropriately trained, and should have the scientific and/or clinical knowledge needed to monitor the trial adequately. A monitor's qualifi-

cations should be documented.

(c) Monitors should be thoroughly familiar with the investigational product(s), the protocol, written informed
consent form and any other written information to be provided to subjects, the sponsor's SOPs, GCP, and the applicable regulatory requirement(s).

5.18.3 *Extent and Nature of Monitoring*

The sponsor should ensure that the trials are adequately monitored. The sponsor should determine the appropriate extent and nature of monitoring. The determination of the extent and nature of monitoring should be based on considerations such as the objective, purpose, design, complexity, blinding, size, and endpoints of the trial. In general there is a need for on-site monitoring, before, during, and after the trial; however in exceptional circumstances the sponsor may determine that central monitoring in conjunction with procedures such as investigators' training and meetings, and extensive written guidance can assure appropriate conduct of the trial in accordance with GCP. Statistically controlled sampling may be an acceptable method for selecting the data to be verified.

5.18.4 *Monitor's Responsibilities*

The monitor(s) in accordance with the sponsor's requirements should ensure that the trial is conducted and documented properly by carrying out the following activities when relevant and necessary to the trial and the trial site:

(a) Acting as the main line of communication between the sponsor and the investigator.

(b) Verifying that the investigator has adequate qualifications and resources (see 4.1, 4.2, 5.6) and remain adequate throughout the trial period, that facilities, including laboratories, equipment, and staff, are adequate to safely and properly conduct the trial and remain adequate throughout the trial period.

(c) Verifying, for the investigational product(s):

  (i) That storage times and conditions are acceptable, and that supplies are sufficient throughout the trial.

  (ii) That the investigational product(s) are supplied only to subjects who are eligible to receive it and at the protocol specified dose(s).

  (iii) That subjects are provided with necessary instruction on properly using, handling, storing, and returning the investigational product(s).

  (iv) That the receipt, use, and return of the investigational product(s) at the trial sites are controlled and documented adequately.

  (v) That the disposition of unused investigational product(s) at the trial sites complies with applicable regulatory requirement(s) and is in accordance with the sponsor.

(d) Verifying that the investigator follows the approved protocol and all approved amendment(s), if any.

(e) Verifying that written informed consent was obtained before each subject's participation in the trial.

(f) Ensuring that the investigator receives the current Investigator's Brochure, all documents, and all trial supplies needed to conduct the trial properly and to comply with the applicable regulatory requirement(s).

(g) Ensuring that the investigator and the investigator's trial staff are adequately informed about the trial.

(h) Verifying that the investigator and the investigator's trial staff are performing the specified trial functions, in accordance with the protocol and any other written agreement between the sponsor and the investigator/institution, and have not delegated these functions to unauthorized individuals.

(i) Verifying that the investigator is enroling only eligible subjects.

(j) Reporting the subject recruitment rate.

(k) Verifying that source documents

and other trial records are accurate, complete, kept up-to-date and maintained.

(l) Verifying that the investigator provides all the required reports, notifications, applications, and submissions, and that these documents are accurate, complete, timely, legible, dated, and identify the trial.

(m) Checking the accuracy and completeness of the CRF entries, source documents and other trial-related records against each other. The monitor specifically should verify that:

  (i) The data required by the protocol are reported accurately on the CRFs and are consistent with the source documents.

  (ii) Any dose and/or therapy modifications are well documented for each of the trial subjects.

  (iii) Adverse events, concomitant medications and intercurrent illnesses are reported in accordance with the protocol on the CRFs.

  (iv) Visits that the subjects fail to make, tests that are not conducted, and examinations that are not performed are clearly reported as such on the CRFs.

  (v) All withdrawals and dropouts of enrolled subjects from the trial are reported and explained on the CRFs.

(n) Informing the investigator of any CRF entry error, omission, or illegibility. The monitor should ensure that appropriate corrections, additions, or deletions are made, dated, explained (if necessary), and initialled by the investigator or by a member of the investigator's trial staff who is authorized to initial CRF changes for the investigator. This authorization should be documented.

(o) Determining whether all adverse events (AEs) are appropriately reported within the time periods required by GCP, the protocol, the IRB/IEC, the sponsor, and the applicable regulatory requirement(s).

(p) Determining whether the investigator is maintaining the essential documents (see 8. Essential Documents for the Conduct of a Clinical Trial).

(q) Communicating deviations from the protocol, SOPs, GCP, and the applicable regulatory requirements to the investigator and taking appropriate action designed to prevent recurrence of the detected deviations.

5.18.5 *Monitoring Procedures*
The monitor(s) should follow the sponsor's established written SOPs as well as those procedures that are specified by the sponsor for monitoring a specific trial.

5.18.6 *Monitoring Report*

(a) The monitor should submit a written report to the sponsor after each trial-site visit or trial-related communication.

(b) Reports should include the date, site, name of the monitor, and name of the investigator or other individual(s) contacted.

(c) Reports should include a summary of what the monitor reviewed and the monitor's statements concerning the significant findings/facts, deviations and deficiencies, conclusions, actions taken or to be taken and/or actions recommended to secure compliance.

(d) The review and follow-up of the monitoring report with the sponsor should be documented by the sponsor's designated representative.

5.19 Audit

If or when sponsors perform audits, as part of implementing quality assurance, they should consider:

5.19.1 *Purpose*

The purpose of a sponsor's audit, which is independent of and separate from routine monitoring or quality control functions, should be to evaluate trial conduct and compliance with the protocol, SOPs, GCP, and the applicable regulatory requirements.

5.19.2 *Selection and Qualification of Auditors*

(a) The sponsor should appoint individuals, who are independent of the clinical trials/systems, to conduct audits.

(b) The sponsor should ensure that the auditors are qualified by training and experience to conduct audits properly. An auditor's qualifications should be documented.

5.19.3 *Auditing Procedures*

(a) The sponsor should ensure that the auditing of clinical trials/systems is conducted in accordance with the sponsor's written procedures on what to audit, how to audit, the frequency of audits, and the form and content of audit reports.

(b) The sponsor's audit plan and procedures for a trial audit should be guided by the importance of the trial to submissions to regulatory authorities, the number of subjects in the trial, the type and complexity of the trial, the level of risks to the trial subjects, and any identified problem(s).

(c) The observations and findings of the auditor(s) should be documented.

(d) To preserve the independence and value of the audit function, the regulatory authority(ies) should not routinely request the audit reports. Regulatory authority(ies) may seek access to an audit report on a case by case basis when evidence of serious GCP non-compliance exists, or in the course of legal proceedings.

(e) When required by applicable law or regulation, the sponsor should provide an audit certificate.

5.20 Noncompliance

5.20.1 Noncompliance with the protocol, SOPs, GCP, and/or applicable regulatory requirement(s) by an investigator/institution, or by member(s) of the sponsor's staff should lead to prompt action by the sponsor to secure compliance.

5.20.2 If the monitoring and/or auditing identifies serious and/or persistent noncompliance on the part of an investigator/institution, the sponsor should terminate the investigator's/institution's participation in the trial. When an investigator's/institution's participation is terminated because of noncompliance, the sponsor should notify promptly the regulatory authority(ies).

5.21 Premature Termination or Suspension of a Trial

If a trial is prematurely terminated or suspended, the sponsor should promptly inform the investigators/institutions, and the regulatory authority(ies) of the termination or suspension and the reason(s) for the termination or suspension. The

IRB/IEC should also be informed promptly and provided the reason(s) for the termination or suspension by the sponsor or by the investigator/institution, as specified by the applicable regulatory requirement(s).

5.22 Clinical Trial/Study Reports

Whether the trial is completed or prematurely terminated, the sponsor should ensure that the clinical trial reports are prepared and provided to the regulatory agency(ies) as required by the applicable regulatory requirement(s). The sponsor should also ensure that the clinical trial reports in marketing applications meet the standards of the ICH Guideline for Structure and Content of Clinical Study Reports. (NOTE: The ICH Guideline for Structure and Content of Clinical Study Reports specifies that abbreviated study reports may be acceptable in certain cases.)

5.23 Multicentre Trials

For multicentre trials, the sponsor should ensure that:

5.23.1 All investigators conduct the trial in strict compliance with the protocol agreed to by the sponsor and, if required, by the regulatory authority(ies), and given approval/favourable opinion by the IRB/IEC.

5.23.2 The CRFs are designed to capture the required data at all multicentre trial sites. For those investigators who are collecting additional data, supplemental CRFs should also be provided that are designed to capture the additional data.

5.23.3 The responsibilities of coordinating investigator(s) and the other participating investigators are documented prior to the start of the trial.

5.23.4 All investigators are given instructions on following the protocol, on complying with a uniform set of standards for the assessment of clinical and laboratory findings, and on completing the CRFs.

5.23.5 Communication between investigators is facilitated.

6. CLINICAL TRIAL PROTOCOL AND PROTOCOL AMENDMENT(S)

The contents of a trial protocol should generally include the following topics. However, site specific information may be provided on separate protocol page(s), or addressed in a separate agreement, and some of the information listed below may be contained in other protocol referenced documents, such as an Investigator's Brochure.

6.1 General Information

6.1.1 Protocol title, protocol identifying number, and date. Any amendment(s) should also bear the amendment number(s) and date(s).

6.1.2 Name and address of the sponsor and monitor (if other than the sponsor).

6.1.3 Name and title of the person(s) authorized to sign the protocol and the protocol amendment(s) for the sponsor.

6.1.4 Name, title, address, and telephone number(s) of the sponsor's medical expert (or dentist when appropriate) for the trial.

6.1.5 Name and title of the investigator(s) who is (are) responsible for conducting the trial, and the address and telephone number(s) of the trial site(s).

6.1.6 Name, title, address, and telephone number(s) of the qualified physician (or dentist, if applicable), who is responsible for all trial-site related medical (or dental) decisions (if other than investigator).

6.1.7 Name(s) and address(es) of the clinical laboratory(ies) and other medical and/or technical department(s) and/or institutions involved in the trial.

6.2 Background Information

6.2.1 Name and description of the investigational product(s).

6.2.2 A summary of findings from nonclinical studies that potentially have clinical significance and from clinical trials that are relevant to the trial.

6.2.3 Summary of the known and potential risks and benefits, if any, to human subjects.

6.2.4 Description of and justification for the route of administration, dosage, dosage regimen, and treatment period(s).

6.2.5 A statement that the trial will be conducted in compliance with the protocol, GCP and the applicable regulatory requirement(s).

6.2.6 Description of the population to be studied.

6.2.7 References to literature and data that are relevant to the trial, and that provide background for the trial.

6.3 Trial Objectives and Purpose
A detailed description of the objectives and the purpose of the trial.

6.4 Trial Design
The scientific integrity of the trial and the credibility of the data from the trial depend substantially on the trial design. A description of the trial design, should include:

6.4.1 A specific statement of the primary endpoints and the secondary endpoints, if any, to be measured during the trial.

6.4.2 A description of the type/design of trial to be conducted (eg. double-blind, placebo-controlled, parallel design) and a schematic diagram of trial design, procedures and stages.

6.4.3 A description of the measures taken to minimize/avoid bias, including:
(a) Randomization.
(b) Blinding.

6.4.4 A description of the trial treatment(s) and the dosage and dosage regimen of the investigational product(s). Also include a description of the dosage form, packaging, and labelling of the investigational product(s).

6.4.5 The expected duration of subject participation, and a description of the sequence and duration of all trial periods, including follow-up, if any.

6.4.6 A description of the "stopping rules" or "discontinuation criteria" for individual subjects, parts of trial and entire trial.

6.4.7 Accountability procedures for the investigational product(s), including the placebo(s) and comparator(s), if any.

6.4.8 Maintenance of trial treatment randomization codes and procedures for breaking codes.

6.4.9 The identification of any data to be recorded directly on the CRFs (ie. no prior written or electronic record of data), and to be considered to be source data.

6.5 Selection and Withdrawal of Subjects
6.5.1 Subject inclusion criteria.

6.5.2 Subject exclusion criteria.

6.5.3 Subject withdrawal criteria (ie. terminating investigational product treatment/trial treatment) and procedures specifying:

(a) When and how to withdraw subjects from the trial/investigational product treatment.

(b) The type and timing of the data to be collected for withdrawn subjects.

(c) Whether and how subjects are to be replaced.

(d) The follow-up for subjects withdrawn from investigational product treatment/trial treatment.

6.6 Treatment of Subjects

6.6.1 The treatment(s) to be administered, including the name(s) of all the product(s), the dose(s), the dosing schedule(s), the route/mode(s) of administration, and the treatment period(s), including the follow-up period(s) for subjects for each investigational product treatment/trial treatment group/arm of the trial.

6.6.2 Medication(s)/treatment(s) permitted (including rescue medication) and not permitted before and/or during the trial.

6.6.3 Procedures for monitoring subject compliance.

6.7 Assessment of Efficacy

6.7.1 Specification of the efficacy parameters.

6.7.2 Methods and timing for assessing, recording, and analysing of efficacy parameters.

6.8 Assessment of Safety

6.8.1 Specification of safety parameters.

6.8.2 The methods and timing for assessing, recording, and analysing safety parameters.

6.8.3 Procedures for eliciting reports of and for recording and reporting adverse event and intercurrent illnesses.

6.8.4 The type and duration of the follow-up of subjects after adverse events.

6.9 Statistics

6.9.1 A description of the statistical methods to be employed, including timing of any planned interim analysis(ses).

6.9.2 The number of subjects planned to be enrolled. In multicentre trials, the numbers of enrolled subjects projected for each trial site should be specified. Reason for choice of sample size, including reflections on (or calculations of) the power of the trial and clinical justification.

6.9.3 The level of significance to be used.

6.9.4 Criteria for the termination of the trial.

6.9.5 Procedure for accounting for

missing, unused, and spurious data.

6.9.6 Procedures for reporting any deviation(s) from the original statistical plan (any deviation(s) from the original statistical plan should be described and justified in protocol and/or in the final report, as appropriate).

6.9.7 The selection of subjects to be included in the analyses (eg. all randomized subjects, all dosed subjects, all eligible subjects, evaluable subjects).

6.10 Direct Access to Source Data/Documents
The sponsor should ensure that it is specified in the protocol or other written agreement that the investigator(s)/institution(s) will permit trial-related monitoring, audits, IRB/IEC review, and regulatory inspection(s), providing direct access to source data/documents.

6.11 Quality Control and Quality Assurance

6.12 Ethics
Description of ethical considerations relating to the trial.

6.13 Data Handling and Record Keeping

6.14 Financing and Insurance
Financing and insurance if not addressed in a separate agreement.

6.15 Publication Policy
Publication policy, if not addressed in a separate agreement.

6.16 Supplements
(NOTE: Since the protocol and the clinical trial/study report are closely related, further relevant information can be found in the ICH Guideline for Structure and Content of Clinical Study Reports.)

7. INVESTIGATOR'S BROCHURE

7.1 Introduction

The Investigator's Brochure (IB) is a compilation of the clinical and non-clinical data on the investigational product(s) that are relevant to the study of the product(s) in human subjects. Its purpose is to provide the investigators and others involved in the trial with the information to facilitate their understanding of the rationale for, and their compliance with, many key features of the protocol, such as the dose, dose frequency/interval, methods of administration: and safety monitoring procedures. The IB also provides insight to support the clinical management of the study subjects during the course of the clinical trial. The information should be presented in a concise, simple, objective, balanced, and non-promotional form that enables a clinician, or potential investigator, to understand it and make his/her own unbiased risk-benefit assessment of the appropriateness of the proposed trial. For this reason, a medically qualified person should generally participate in the editing of an IB, but the contents of the IB should be approved by the disciplines that generated the described data.

This guideline delineates the minimum information that should be included in an IB and provides suggestions for its layout. It is expected that the type and extent of information available will vary with the stage of development of the investigational product. If the investigational product is marketed and its pharmacology is widely understood by medical practitioners, an extensive IB may not be necessary. Where permitted by regulatory authorities, a basic product information brochure, package leaflet, or labelling may be an appropriate alternative, provided that it includes current, comprehensive, and detailed information on all aspects of the investigational product that might be of importance to the investigator. If a marketed product is being studied for a new use (ie., a new indication), an IB specific to that new use should be prepared. The IB should be reviewed at least annually and revised as necessary in compliance with a sponsor's written procedures. More frequent revision may be appropriate depending on the stage of development and the generation of relevant new information. However, in accordance with Good Clinical Practice, relevant new information may be so important that it should be communicated to the investigators, and possibly to the Institutional Review Boards (IRBs)/ Independent Ethics Committees (IECs) and/or regulatory authorities before it is included in a revised IB.

Generally, the sponsor is responsible for ensuring that an up-to-date IB is made available to the investigator(s) and the investigators are responsible for providing the up-to-date IB to the responsible IRBs/IECs. In the case of an investigator sponsored trial, the sponsor-investigator should determine whether a brochure is available from the commercial manufacturer. If the investigational product is provided by the sponsor-investigator, then he or she should provide the necessary information to the trial personnel. In cases where preparation of a formal IB is impractical, the sponsor-investigator should provide, as a substitute, an expanded background information section in the trial protocol that contains the minimum current information described in this guideline.

7.2 General Considerations
The IB should include:

7.2.1 *Title Page*
This should provide the sponsor's name, the identity of each investigational product (ie. research number, chemical or approved generic name, and trade name(s) where legally permissible and desired by the sponsor), and the release date. It is also suggested that an edition number, and a reference to the number and date of the edition it supersedes, be provided. An example is given in Appendix I.

7.2.2 *Confidentiality Statement*
The sponsor may wish to include a statement instructing the investigator/recipients to treat the IB as a confidential document for the sole information and use of the investigator's team and the IRB/IEC.

7.3 Contents of the Investigator's Brochure
The IB should contain the following sections, each with literature references where appropriate:

7.3.1 *Table of Contents*
An example of the Table of Contents is given in Appendix 2

7.3.2 *Summary*
A brief summary (preferably not exceeding two pages) should be given, highlighting the significant physical, chemical, pharmaceutical, pharmacological, toxicological, pharmacokinetic, metabolic, and clinical information available that is relevant to the stage of clinical development of the investigational product.

7.3.3 *Introduction*
A brief introductory statement should be provided that contains the chemical name (and generic and trade name(s) when approved) of the investigational product(s), all active ingredients, the investigational product(s) pharmacological class and its expected position within this class (eg. advantages), the rationale for performing research with the investigational product(s), and the anticipated prophylactic, therapeutic, or diagnostic indication(s). Finally, the introductory statement should

provide the general approach to be followed in evaluating the investigational product.

7.3.4 *Physical, Chemical, and Pharmaceutical Properties and Formulation*
A description should be provided of the investigational product substance(s) (including the chemical and/or structural formula(e)), and a brief summary should be given of the relevant physical, chemical, and pharmaceutical properties.

To permit appropriate safety measures to be taken in the course of the trial, a description of the formulation(s) to be used, including excipients, should be provided and justified if clinically relevant. Instructions for the storage and handling of the dosage form(s) should also be given.

Any structural similarities to other known compounds should be mentioned.

7.3.5 *Nonclinical Studies*
Introduction:
The results of all relevant nonclinical pharmacology, toxicology, pharmacokinetic, and investigational product metabolism studies should be provided in summary form. This summary should address the methodology used, the results, and a discussion of the relevance of the findings to the investigated therapeutic and the possible unfavourable and unintended effects in humans.

The information provided may include the following, as appropriate, if known/available:
- Species tested
- Number and sex of animals in each group
- Unit dose (eg. milligram/kilogram (mg/kg))
- Dose interval
- Route of administration
- Duration of dosing
- Information on systemic distribution
- Duration of post-exposure follow-up
- Results, including the following aspects:
  - Nature and frequency of pharmacological or toxic effects
  - Severity or intensity of pharmacological or toxic effects
  - Time to onset of effects
  - Reversibility of effects
  - Duration of effects
  - Dose response

Tabular format/listings should be used whenever possible to enhance the clarity of the presentation.

The following sections should discuss the most important findings from the studies, including the dose response of observed effects, the relevance to humans, and any aspects to be studied in humans. If applicable, the effective and nontoxic dose findings in the same animal species should be compared (ie. the therapeutic index should be discussed). The relevance of this information to the proposed human dosing should be addressed. Whenever possible, comparisons should be made in terms of blood/tissue levels rather than on a mg/kg basis.

(a) Nonclinical Pharmacology
A summary of the pharmacological aspects of the investigational product and, where appropriate, its significant metabolites studied in animals, should be included. Such a summary should incorporate studies that assess potential therapeutic activity (eg. efficacy models, receptor binding, and specificity) as well as those that assess safety (eg. special studies to assess pharmacological actions other than the intended therapeutic effect(s)).

(b) Pharmacokinetics and Product Metabolism in Animals
A summary of the pharmacokinetics and biological transformation and disposition of the investigational product in all species studied should be given. The discussion of the findings should address the absorption and the local and systemic bioavailability of the investigational product and its meta-bolites, and their relationship to the pharmacological and toxicological findings in animal species.

(c) Toxicology
A summary of the toxicological effects found in relevant studies conducted in different animal species

should be described under the following headings where appropriate:
- Single dose
- Repeated dose
- Carcinogenicity
- Special studies (eg. irritancy and sensitisation)
- Reproductive toxicity
- Genotoxicity (mutagenicity)

7.3.6 *Effects in Humans*
Introduction:
A thorough discussion of the known effects of the investigational product(s) in humans should be provided, including information on pharmacokinetics, metabolism, pharmacodynamics, dose response, safety, efficacy, and other pharmacological activities. Where possible, a summary of each completed clinical trial should be provided. Information should also be provided regarding results of any use of the investigational product(s) other than from in clinical trials, such as from experience during marketing.

(a) Pharmacokinetics and Product Metabolism in Humans
- A summary of information on the pharmacokinetics of the investigational product(s) should be presented, including the following, if available:
- Pharmacokinetics (including metabolism, as appropriate, and absorption, plasma protein binding, distribution, and elimination).
- Bioavailability of the investiga-

tional product (absolute, where possible, and/or relative) using a reference dosage form.

- Population subgroups (eg. gender, age, and impaired organ function).
- Interactions (eg. product-product interactions and effects of food).
- Other pharmacokinetic data (eg. results of population studies performed within clinical trial(s).

(b) Safety and Efficacy
A summary of information should be provided about the investigational product's/products' (including metabolites, where appropriate) safety, pharmacodynamics, efficacy, and dose response that were obtained from preceding trials in humans (healthy volunteers and/or patients). The implications of this information should be discussed. In cases where a number of clinical trials have been completed, the use of summaries of safety and efficacy across multiple trials by indications in subgroups may provide a clear presentation of the data. Tabular summaries of adverse drug reactions for all the clinical trials (including those for all the studied indications) would be useful. Important differences in adverse drug reaction patterns/incidences across indications or subgroups should be discussed.

The IB should provide a description of the possible risks and adverse

drug reactions to be anticipated on the basis of prior experiences with the product under investigation and with related products. A description should also be provided of the precautions or special monitoring to be done as part of the investigational use of the product(s).

(c) Marketing Experience
The IB should identify countries where the investigational product has been marketed or approved. Any significant information arising from the marketed use should be summarised (eg. formulations, dosages, routes of administration, and adverse product reactions). The IB should also identify all the countries where the investigational product did not receive approval/registration for marketing or was withdrawn from marketing/registration.

7.3.7 *Summary of Data and Guidance for the Investigator*
This section should provide an overall discussion of the nonclinical and clinical data, and should summarise the information from various sources on different aspects of the investigational product(s), wherever possible. In this way, the investigator can be provided with the most informative interpretation of the available data and with an assessment of the implications of the information for future clinical trials.

Where appropriate, the published

reports on related products should be discussed. This could help the investigator to anticipate adverse drug reactions or other problems in clinical trials.

The overall aim of this section is to provide the investigator with a clear understanding of the possible risks and adverse reactions, and of the specific tests, observations, and precautions that may be needed for a clinical trial. This understanding should be based on the available physical, chemical, pharmaceutical, pharmacological, toxicological, and clinical information on the investigational product(s). Guidance should also be provided to the clinical investigator on the recognition and treatment of possible overdose and adverse drug reactions that is based on previous human experience and on the pharmacology of the investigational product.

7.4 APPENDIX 1:

TITLE PAGE *(Example)*
SPONSOR'S NAME
Product:
Research Number:
Name(s): Chemical, Generic
           (if approved)
           Trade Name(s) (if legally
           permissible and desired
           by the sponsor)

INVESTIGATOR'S BROCHURE
Edition Number:

Release Date:
Replaces Previous Edition Number:
Date:

7.5 APPENDIX 2:

TABLE OF CONTENTS OF INVESTIGATOR'S BROCHURE *(Example)*

– Confidentiality Statement (optional)
– Signature Page (optional)
I   Table of Contents
2   Summary
3   Introduction
4   Physical, Chemical, and Pharmaceutical Properties and Formulation
5   Nonclinical Studies
    5.1 Nonclinical Pharmacology
    5.2 Pharmacokinetics and Product Metabolism in Animals
    5.3 Toxicology
6   Effects in Humans
    6.1 Pharmacokinetics and Product Metabolism in Humans
    6.2 Safety and Efficacy
    6.3 Marketing Experience
7   Summary of Data and Guidance for the Investigator

NB: References on   1. Publications
                    2. Reports

These references should be found at the end of each chapter

Appendices (if any)

8. ESSENTIAL DOCUMENTS FOR THE CONDUCT OF A CLINICAL TRIAL

8.1 Introduction

Essential Documents are those documents which individually and collectively permit evaluation of the conduct of a trial and the quality of the data produced. These documents serve to demonstrate the compliance of the investigator, sponsor and monitor with the standards of Good Clinical Practice and with all applicable regulatory requirements.

Essential Documents also serve a number of other important purposes. Filing essential documents at the investigator/institution and sponsor sites in a timely manner can greatly assist in the successful management of a trial by the investigator, sponsor and monitor. These documents are also the ones which are usually audited by the sponsor's independent audit function and inspected by the regulatory authority(ies) as part of the process to confirm the validity of the trial conduct and the integrity of data collected.

The minimum list of essential documents which has been developed follows. The various documents are grouped in three sections according to the stage of the trial during which they will normally be generated:

1) before the clinical phase of the trial commences, 2) during the clinical conduct of the trial, and 3) after completion or termination of the trial. A description is given of the purpose of each document, and whether it should be filed in either the investigator/institution or sponsor files, or both. It is acceptable to combine some of the documents, provided the individual elements are readily identifiable.

Trial master files should be established at the beginning of the trial, both at the investigator/institution's site and at the sponsor's office. A final close-out of a trial can only be done when the monitor has reviewed both investigator/institution and sponsor files and confirmed that all necessary documents are in the appropriate files.

Any or all of the documents addressed in this guideline may be subject to, and should be available for, audit by the sponsor's auditor and inspection by the regulatory authority(ies).

Title of Document	Purpose	Located in Files of	
		Investigator/ Institution	Sponsor

8.2 Before the Clinical Phase of the Trial Commences

During this planning stage the following documents should be generated and should be on file before the trial formally starts

Title of Document	Purpose	Located in Files of Investigator/ Institution	Sponsor
8.2.1 INVESTIGATOR'S BROCHURE	To document that relevant and current scientific information about the investigational product has been provided to the investigator	X	X
8.2.2 SIGNED PROTOCOL AND AMENDMENTS, IF ANY, AND SAMPLE CASE REPORT FORM (CRF)	To document investigator and sponsor agreement to the protocol/ amendment(s) and CRF	X	X
8.2.3 INFORMATION GIVEN TO TRIAL SUBJECT – INFORMED CONSENT FORM (including all applicable translations)	To document the informed consent	X	X
– ANY OTHER WRITTEN INFORMATION	To document that subjects will be given appropriate written information (content and wording) to support their ability to give fully informed consent	X	X
– ADVERTISEMENT FOR SUBJECT RECRUITMENT (if used)	To document that recruitment measures are appropriate and not coercive	X	
8.2.4 FINANCIAL ASPECTS OF THE TRIAL	To document the financial agreement between the investigator/institution and the sponsor for the trial	X	X

| Title of Document | Purpose | Located in Files of | |
		Investigator/ Institution	Sponsor
8.2.5 INSURANCE STATEMENT (where required)	To document that compensation to subject(s) for trial-related injury will be available	X	X
8.2.6 SIGNED AGREEMENT BETWEEN INVOLVED PARTIES, eg.:	To document agreements		
– investigator/institution and sponsor		X	X
– investigator/institution and CRO		X	X (where required)
– sponsor and CRO			X
– investigator/institution and authority(ies) (where required)		X	X
8.2.7 DATED, DOCU-MENTED APPROVAL/ FAVOURABLE OPINION OF INSTI-TUTIONAL REVIEW BOARD (IRB)/INDE-PENDENT ETHICS COMMITTEE (IEC) OF THE FOLLOWING: – protocol and any amendments – CRF (if applicable) – informed consent form(s) – any other written information to be provided to the subject(s) – advertisement for subject recruitment (if used) – subject compensa-	To document that the trial has been subject to IRB/IEC review and given approval/favourable opinion. To identify the version number and date of the document(s)	X	X

Title of Document	Purpose	Located in Files of	
		Investigator/ Institution	Sponsor
tion (if any) – any other docu- ments given approval/favourable opinion			
8.2.8 INSTITUTIONAL REVIEW BOARD/ INDEPENDENT ETHICS COMMITTEE COMPOSITION	To document that the IRB/IEC is constituted in agreement with GCP	X	X (where required)
8.2.9 REGULATORY AUTHORITY(IES) AUTHORISATION/ APPROVAL/ NOTIFI-CATION OF PROTO-COL (where required)	To document appropriate authorisation/approval/ notifi-cation by the regulatory authority(ies) has been obtained prior to initiation of the trial in compliance with the applicable regulatory requirement(s)	X (where required)	X (where required)
8.2.10 CURRICULUM VITAE AND/OR OTHER RELEVANT DOCU-MENTS EVIDENCING QUALIFICATIONS OF INVESTIGATOR(S) AND SUB-INVESTIGATOR(S)	To document qualifications and eligibility to conduct trial and/or provide medical supervision of subjects	X	X
8.2.11 NORMAL VALUE(S) /RANGE(S) FOR MEDICAL/ LABORA-TORY/TECHNICAL PROCEDURE(S) AND/OR TEST(S) INCLUDED IN THE PROTOCOL	To document normal values and/or ranges of the tests	X	X

Title of Document	Purpose	Located in Files of Investigator/ Institution	Sponsor
8.2.12 MEDICAL/LABORA-TORY/TECHNICAL PROCEDURES/TESTS – certification or – accreditation or – established quality control and/or external quality assessment or – other validation (where required)	To document competence of facility to perform required test(s), and support reliability of results	X (where required)	X
8.2.13 SAMPLE OF LABEL(S) ATTACHED TO INVESTIGATIONAL PRODUCT CONTAINER(S)	To document compliance with applicable labelling regulations and appropriate-ness of instructions provided to the subjects		X
8.2.14 INSTRUCTIONS FOR HANDLING OF INVESTIGATIONAL PRODUCT(S) AND TRIAL-RELATED MATERIALS (if not included in protocol or Investigator's Brochure)	To document instructions needed to ensure proper storage, packaging, dispensing and disposition of investiga-tional products and trial-related materials	X	X
8.2.15 SHIPPING RECORDS FOR INVESTIGA-TIONAL PROD-UCT(S) AND TRIAL-RELATED MATERIALS	To document shipment dates, batch numbers and method of shipment of inves-tigational product(s) and trial-related materials. Allows tracking of product batch, review of shipping conditions, and accountability	X	X

Title of Document	Purpose	Located in Files of	
		Investigator/ Institution	Sponsor
8.2.16 CERTIFICATE(S) OF ANALYSIS OF INVESTIGATIONAL PRODUCT(S) SHIPPED	To document identity, purity, and strength of investigational product(s) to be used in the trial		X
8.2.17 DECODING PROCEDURES FOR BLINDED TRIALS	To document how, in case of an emergency, identity of blinded investigational product can be revealed without breaking the blind for the remaining subjects' treatment	X	X (third party if applicable)
8.2.18 MASTER RANDOMI-SATION LIST	To document method for randomisation of trial population		X (third party if applicable)
8.2.19 PRE-TRIAL MONI-TORING REPORT	To document that the site is suitable for the trial (may be combined with 8.2.20)		X
8.2.20 TRIAL INITIATION MONITORING REPORT	To document that trial procedures were reviewed with the investigator and the investigator's trial staff (may be combined with 8.2.19)	X	X

8.3 During the Clinical Conduct of the Trial

In addition to having on file the above documents, the following should be added to the files during the trial as evidence that all new relevant information is documented as it becomes available

8.3.1 INVESTIGATOR'S BROCHURE UPDATES	To document that investigator is informed in a timely manner of relevant information as it becomes available	X	X

Title of Document	Purpose	Located in Files of	
		Investigator/ Institution	Sponsor
8.3.2 ANY REVISION TO: – protocol/amend ment(s) and CRF – informed consent form – any other written information provided to subjects – advertisement for subject recruit- ment(if used)	To document revisions of these trial related documents that take effect during trial	X	X

8.3.3 DATED, DOCU- MENTED APPROVAL/FAVOUR- ABLE OPINION OF INSTITUTIONAL REVIEW BOARD (IRB)/INDEPENDENT ETHICS COMMITTEE (IEC) OF THE FOLLOWING:
 – protocol amend ment(s)
 – revision(s) of:
    – informed consent form
    – any other written information to be provided to the subject
    – advertisement for subject recruitment (if used)
 – any other documents
	To document that the amendment(s) and/or revi- sion(s) have been subject to IRB/IEC review and were given approval/favourable opinion. To identify the ver- sion number and date of the document(s).	X	X

Title of Document	Purpose	Located in Files of Investigator/ Institution	Sponsor
given approval/ favourable opinion – continuing review of trial (where required)			
8.3.4 REGULATORY AUTHORITY(IES) AUTHORISATIONS/ APPROVALS/NOTIFI-CATIONS WHERE REQUIRED FOR: – protocol amend ment(s) and other documents	To document compliance with applicable regulatory requirements	X (where required)	X
8.3.5 CURRICULUM VITAE FOR NEW INVESTIGATOR(S) AND/OR SUB-INVESTIGATOR(S)	(see 8.2.10)	X	X
8.3.6 UPDATES TO NOR-MAL VALUE(S)/ RANGE(S) FOR MEDICAL/LABORA-TORY/TECHNICAL PROCEDURE(S)/ TEST(S) INCLUDED IN THE PROTOCOL	To document normal values and ranges that are revised during the trial (see 8.2.11)	X	X
8.3.7 UPDATES OF MEDICAL/ LABORA-TORY/TECHNICAL PROCEDURES/ TESTS – certification or – accreditation or	To document that tests remain adequate throughout the trial period (see 8.2.12)	X (where required)	X

Title of Document	Purpose	Located in Files of	
		Investigator/ Institution	Sponsor
– established quality control and/or external quality assessment or – other validation (where required)			
8.3.8 DOCUMENTATION OF INVESTIGA-TIONAL PROD-UCT(S) AND TRIAL-RELATED MATERI-ALS SHIPMENT	(see 8.2.15)	X	X
8.3.9 CERTIFICATE(S) OF ANALYSIS FOR NEW BATCHES OF INVESTIGATIONAL PRODUCTS	(see 8.2.16)		X
8.3.10 MONITORING VISIT REPORTS	To document site visits by, and findings of, the monitor		X

8.3.11 RELEVANT COMMUNICATIONS OTHER THAN SITE VISITS
    – letters
    – meeting notes
    – notes of telephone calls
	To document any agree-ments or significant discus-sions regarding trial adminis-tration, protocol violations, trial conduct, adverse event (AE) reporting	X	X

8.3.12 SIGNED INFORMED CONSENT FORMS	To document that consent is obtained in accordance with GCP and protocol and dated prior to participation of each subject in trial. Also to docu-ment direct access permis-sion (see 8.2.3)	X	

Title of Document	Purpose	Located in Files of Investigator/ Institution	Sponsor
8.3.13 SOURCE DOCUMENTS	To document the existence of the subject and substantiate integrity of trial data collected. To include original documents related to the trial, to medical treatment, and history of subject	X	
8.3.14 SIGNED, DATED AND COMPLETED CASE REPORT FORMS (CRF)	To document that the investigator or authorised member of the investigator's staff confirms the observations recorded	X (copy)	X (original)
8.3.15 DOCUMENTATION OF CRF CORRECTIONS	To document all changes/additions or corrections made to CRF after initial data were recorded	X (copy)	X (original)
8.3.16 NOTIFICATION BY ORIGINATING INVESTIGATOR TO SPONSOR OF SERIOUS ADVERSE EVENTS AND RELATED REPORTS	Notification by originating investigator to sponsor of serious adverse events and related reports in accordance with 4.11	X	X
8.3.17 NOTIFICATION BY SPONSOR AND/OR INVESTIGATOR, WHERE APPLICABLE, TO REGULATORY AUTHORITY(IES) AND IRB(S)/IEC(S) OF UNEXPECTED SERIOUS ADVERSE DRUG REACTIONS AND OF OTHER SAFETY INFORMATION	Notification by sponsor and/or investigator, where applicable, to regulatory authorities and IRB(s)/ IEC(s) of unexpected serious adverse drug reactions in accordance with 5.17 and 4.11.1 and of other safety information in accordance with 5.16.2	X (where required)	X

Title of Document	Purpose	Located in Files of	
		Investigator/ Institution	Sponsor
8.3.18 NOTIFICATION BY SPONSOR TO INVESTIGATORS OF SAFETY INFORMA-TION	Notification by sponsor to investigators of safety information in accordance with 5.16.2	X	X
8.3.19 INTERIM OR ANNU-AL REPORTS TO IRB/IEC AND AUTHORITY(IES)	Interim or annual reports provided to IRB/IEC in accor-dance with 4.10 and to authority(ies) in accordance with 5.17.3	X	X (where required)
8.3.20 SUBJECT SCREENING LOG	To document identification of subjects who entered pre-trial screening	X	X (where required)
8.3.21 SUBJECT IDENTIFI-CATION CODE LIST	To document that investiga-tor/institution keeps a confi-dential list of names of all subjects allocated to trial numbers on enrolling in the trial. Allows investigator/ institution to reveal identity of any subject	X	
8.3.22 SUBJECT ENROL-MENT LOG	To document chronological enrolment of subjects by trial number	X	
8.3.23 INVESTIGATIONAL PRODUCTS ACCOUNTABILITY AT THE SITE	To document that investiga-tional product(s) have been used according to the protocol	X	X
8.3.24 SIGNATURE SHEET	To document signatures and initials of all persons autho-rised to make entries and/or corrections on CRFs	X	X

Title of Document	Purpose	Located in Files of	
		Investigator/ Institution	Sponsor
8.3.25 RECORD OF RETAINED BODY FLUIDS/TISSUE SAMPLES (IF ANY)	To document location and identification of retained samples if assays need to be repeated	X	X

8.4 After Completion or Termination of the Trial

After completion or termination of the trial, all of the documents identified in sections 8.2 and 8.3 should be in the file together with the following

Title of Document	Purpose	Located in Files of	
		Investigator/ Institution	Sponsor
8.4.1 INVESTIGATIONAL PRODUCT(S) ACCOUNTABILITY AT SITE	To document that the investigational product(s) have been used according to the protocol. To documents the final accounting of investigational product(s) received at the site, dispensed to subjects, returned by the subjects, and returned to sponsor	X	X
8.4.2 DOCUMENTATION OF INVESTIGATIONAL PRODUCT DESTRUCTION	To document destruction of unused investigational products by sponsor or at site	X (if destroyed at site)	X
8.4.3 COMPLETED SUBJECT IDENTIFICATION CODE LIST	To permit identification of all subjects enrolled in the trial in case follow-up is required. List should be kept in a confidential manner and for agreed upon time	X	
8.4.4 AUDIT CERTIFICATE (if available)	To document that audit was performed		X
8.4.5 FINAL TRIAL CLOSE-OUT MONITORING REPORT	To document that all activities required for trial close-out are completed, and copies of essential documents are held in the appropriate files		X

Title of Document	Purpose	Located in Files of	
		Investigator/ Institution	Sponsor
8.4.6 TREATMENT ALLO-CATION AND DECODING DOCU-MENTATION	Returned to sponsor to doc-ument any decoding that may have occurred		X
8.4.7 FINAL REPORT BY INVESTIGATOR TO IRB/IEC WHERE REQUIRED, AND WHERE APPLICA-BLE, TO THE REGU-LATORY AUTHORI-TY(IES)	To document completion of the trial	X	
8.4.8 CLINICAL STUDY REPORT	To document results and interpretation of trial	X (if applicable)	X

Declaration of Helsinki

Ethical principles for medical research involving human subjects

Adopted by the 18th WMA General Assembly, Helsinki, Finland, June 1964, and amended by the 29th WMA General Assembly, Tokyo, Japan, October 1975, 35th WMA General Assembly, Venice, Italy, October 1983 41st WMA General Assembly, Hong Kong, September 1989 48th WMA General Assembly, Somerset West, Republic of South Africa, October 1996 and the 52nd WMA General Assembly, Edinburgh, Scotland, October 2000

A. Introduction

1. The World Medical Association has developed the Declaration of Helsinki as a statement of ethical principles to provide guidance to physicians and other participants in medical research involving human subjects. Medical research involving human subjects includes research on identifiable human material or identifiable data.

2. It is the duty of the physician to promote and safeguard the health of the people. The physician's knowledge and conscience are dedicated to the fulfilment of this duty.

3. The Declaration of Geneva of the World Medical Association binds the physician with the words, "The health of my patient will be my first consideration," and the International Code of Medical Ethics declares that, "A physician shall act only in the patient's interest when providing medical care which might have the effect of weakening the physical and mental condition of the patient."

4. Medical progress is based on research which ultimately must rest in part on experimentation involving human subjects.

5. In medical research on human subjects, considerations related to the well-being of the human subject should take precedence over the interests of science and society.

6. The primary purpose of medical research involving human subjects is to improve prophylactic, diagnostic and therapeutic procedures and the understanding of the aetiology and pathogenesis of disease. Even the best proven prophylactic, diagnostic and therapeutic methods must continuously be challenged through research for their effectiveness, efficiency, accessibility and quality.

7. In current medical practice and in medical research, most prophylactic, diagnostic and therapeutic procedures involve risks and burdens.

8. Medical research is subject to

ethical standards that promote respect for all human beings and protect their health and rights. Some research populations are vulnerable and need special protection. The particular needs of the economically and medically disadvantaged must be recognized. Special attention is also required for those who cannot give or refuse consent for themselves, for those who may be subject to giving consent under duress, for those who will not benefit personally from the research and for those for whom the research is combined with care.

9. Research Investigators should be aware of the ethical, legal and regulatory requirements for research on human subjects in their own countries as well as applicable international requirements. No national ethical, legal or regulatory requirement should be allowed to reduce or eliminate any of the protections for human subjects set forth in this Declaration.

B. Basic Principles for all medical research

10. It is the duty of the physician in medical research to protect the life, health, privacy, and dignity of the human subject.

11. Medical research involving human subjects must conform to generally accepted scientific principles, be based on a thorough knowledge of the scientific literature, other relevant sources of information, and on adequate laboratory and, where appropriate, animal experimentation.

12. Appropriate caution must be exercised in the conduct of research which may affect the environment, and the welfare of animals used for research must be respected.

13. The design and performance of each experimental procedure involving human subjects should be clearly formulated in an experimental protocol. This protocol should be submitted for consideration, comment, guidance and, where appropriate, approval to a specially appointed ethical review committee, which must be independent of the investigator, the sponsor or any other kind of undue influence. This independent committee should be in conformity with the laws and regulations of the country in which the research experiment is performed. The committee has the right and obligation to monitor ongoing trials. The researcher has the obligation to provide monitoring information to the committee, especially any serious adverse events. The researcher should

also submit to the committee, for review, information regarding funding, sponsors, institutional affiliations, other potential conflicts of interest and incentives for subjects.

14. The research protocol should always contain a statement of the ethical considerations involved and should indicate that there is compliance with the principles enunciated in this Declaration.

15. Medical research involving human subjects should be conducted only by scientifically qualified persons and under the supervision of a clinically competent medical person. The responsibility for the human subject must always rest with a medically qualified person and never rest on the subject of the research, even though the subject has given consent.

16. Every medical research project involving human subjects should be preceded by careful assessment of predictable risks and burdens in comparison with foreseeable benefits to the subject or to others. This does not preclude the participation of healthy volunteers in medical research. The design of all studies should be publicly available.

17. Physicians should abstain from engaging in research projects involving human subjects unless they are confident that the risks involved have been adequately assessed and can be satisfactorily managed. Physicians should cease any investigation if the risks are found to outweigh the potential benefits or if there is conclusive proof of positive and beneficial results.

18. Medical research involving human subjects should only be conducted if the importance of the objective outweighs the inherent risks and burdens to the subject. This is especially important when the human subjects are healthy volunteers.

19. Medical research is only justified if there is a reasonable likelihood that the populations in which the research is carried out stand to benefit from the results of the research.

20. The subjects must be volunteers and informed participants in the research project.

21. The right of research subjects to safeguard their integrity must always be respected. Every precaution should be taken to respect the privacy of the subject, the confidentiality of the patient's information and to minimise the impact of the study on the subject's

physical and mental integrity and on the personality of the subject.

22. In any research on human beings, each potential subject must be adequately informed of the aims, methods, sources of funding, any possible conflicts of interest, institutional affiliations of the researcher, the anticipated benefits and potential risks of the study and the discomfort it may entail. The subject should be informed of the right to abstain from participation in the study or to withdraw consent to participate at any time without reprisal. After ensuring that the subject has understood the information, the physician should then obtain the subject's freely-given informed consent, preferably in writing. If the consent cannot be obtained in writing, the non-written consent must be formally documented and witnessed.

23. When obtaining informed consent for the research project the physician should be particularly cautious if the subject is in a dependent relationship with the physician or may consent under duress. In that case the informed consent should be obtained by a well-informed physician who is not engaged in the investigation and who is completely independent of this relationship.

24. For a research subject who is legally incompetent, physically or mentally incapable of giving consent or is a legally incompetent minor, the investigator must obtain informed consent from the legally authorised representative in accordance with applicable law. These groups should not be included in research unless the research is necessary to promote the health of the population represented and this research cannot instead be performed on legally competent persons.

25. When a subject deemed legally incompetent, such as a minor child, is able to give assent to decisions about participation in research, the investigator must obtain that assent in addition to the consent of the legally authorised representative.

26. Research on individuals from whom it is not possible to obtain consent, including proxy or advance consent, should be done only if the physical/mental condition that prevents obtaining informed consent is a necessary characteristic of the research population. The specific reasons for involving research subjects with a condition that renders them unable

to give informed consent should be stated in the experimental protocol for consideration and approval of the review committee. The protocol should state that consent to remain in the research should be obtained as soon as possible from the individual or a legally authorised surrogate.

27. Both authors and publishers have ethical obligations. In publication of the results of research, the investigators are obliged to preserve the accuracy of the results. Negative as well as positive results should be published or otherwise publicly available. Sources of funding, institutional affiliations and any possible conflicts of interest should be declared in the publication. Reports of experimentation not in accordance with the principles laid down in this Declaration should not be accepted for publication.

C. Additional Principles For Medical Research Combined With Medical Care

28. The physician may combine medical research with medical care, only to the extent that the research is justified by its potential prophylactic, diagnostic or therapeutic value. When medical research is combined with medical care, additional standards apply to protect the patients who are research subjects.

29. The benefits, risks, burdens and effectiveness of a new method should be tested against those of the best current prophylactic, diagnostic, and therapeutic methods. This does not exclude the use of placebo, or no treatment, in studies where no proven prophylactic, diagnostic or therapeutic method exists.

To further clarifiy the WMA position on the use of placebo controlled trials, the WMA Council issued, during October 2001, a note of clarification on article 29, which is available on page 66.

30. At the conclusion of the study, every patient entered into the study should be assured of access to the best proven prophylactic, diagnostic and therapeutic methods identified by the study.

31. The physician should fully inform the patient which aspects of the care are related to the research. The refusal of a patient to participate in a study must never interfere with the patient-physician relationship.

32. In the treatment of a patient, where proven prophylactic, diagnostic and therapeutic methods do not exist or have been ineffective, the physician, with informed consent from the patient, must be free to use unproven or new prophylactic, diagnostic and therapeutic measures, if in the physician's judgement it offers hope of saving life, re-establishing health or alleviating suffering. Where possible, these measures should be made the object of research, designed to evaluate their safety and efficacy. In all cases, new information should be recorded and, where appropriate, published. The other relevant guidelines of this Declaration should be followed.

NOTE OF CLARIFICATION ON PARAGRAPH 29 of the WMA DECLARATION OF HELSINKI

The WMA is concerned that paragraph 29 of the revised Declaration of Helsinki (October 2000) has led to diverse interpretations and possible confusion. It hereby reaffirms its position that extreme care must be taken in making use of a placebo-controlled trial and that in general this methodology should only be used in the absence of existing proven therapy. However, a placebo-controlled trial may be ethically acceptable, even if proven therapy is available, under the following circumstances:

- Where for compelling and scientifically sound methodological reasons its use is necessary to determine the efficacy or safety of a prophylactic, diagnostic or therapeutic method; or

- Where a prophylactic, diagnostic or therapeutic method is being investigated for a minor condition and the patients who receive placebo will not be subject to any additional risk of serious or irreversible harm.

All other provisions of the Declaration of Helsinki must be adhered to, especially the need for appropriate ethical and scientific review.

DIRECTIVE 2001/20/EC OF THE EUROPEAN PARLIAMENT AND OF THE COUNCIL
of 4 April 2001

on the approximation of the laws, regulations and administrative provisions of the Member States relating to the implementation of good clinical practice in the conduct of clinical trials on medicinal products for human use

THE EUROPEAN PARLIAMENT AND THE COUNCIL OF THE EUROPEAN UNION,

Having regard to the Treaty establishing the European Community, and in particular Article 95 thereof,

Having regard to the proposal from the Commission[1],

Having regard to the opinion of the Economic and Social Committee[2],

Acting in accordance with the procedure laid down in Article 251 of the Treaty[3],

Whereas:

(1) Council Directive 65/65/EEC of 26 January 1965 on the approximation of provisions laid down by law, regulation or administrative action relating to medicinal products[4] requires that applications for authorisation to place a medicinal product on the market should be accompanied by a dossier containing particulars and documents relating to the results of tests and clinical trials carried out on the product. Council Directive 75/318/EEC of

---

[1] OJ C 306,8.10.1997, p.9 and OJ C 161, 8.6.1999, p.5.

[2] OJ C 95, 30.3.1998, p.1.

[3] Opinion of the European Parliament of 17 November 1998 (OJ C 379,7.12.1998, p.27). Council Common Position of 20 July 2000 (OJ C 300, 20.10.2000, p.32) and Decision of the European Parliament of 12 December 2000. Council Decision of 26 February 2001.

[4] (4)OJ 22, 9.2.1965, p.1/65. Directive as last amended by Council Directive 93/39/EEC (OJ L 214, 24.8.1993, p.22).

20 May 1975 on the approximation of the laws of Member States relating to analytical, pharmaco-toxicological and clinical standards and protocols in respect of the testing of medicinal products[1] lays down uniform rules on the compilation of dossiers including their presentation.

(2) The accepted basis for the conduct of clinical trials in humans is founded in the protection of human rights and the dignity of the human being with regard to the application of biology and medicine, as for instance reflected in the 1996 version of the Helsinki Declaration. The clinical trial subject's protection is safeguarded through risk assessment based on the results of toxicological experiments prior to any clinical trial, screening by ethics committees and Member States' competent authorities, and rules on the protection of personal data.

(3) Persons who are incapable of giving legal consent to clinical trials should be given special protection. It is incumbent on the Member States to lay down rules to this effect. Such persons may not be included in clinical trials if the same results can be obtained using persons capable of giving consent. Normally these persons should be included in clinical trials only when there are grounds for expecting that the administering of the medicinal product would be of direct benefit to the patient, thereby outweighing the risks. However, there is a need for clinical trials involving children to improve the treatment available to them. Children represent a vulnerable population with developmental, physiological and psychological differences from adults, which make age- and development-related research important for their benefit. Medicinal products, including vaccines, for children need to be tested scientifically before widespread use. This can only be achieved by ensuring that medicinal products which are likely to be of significant clinical value for children are fully studied. The clinical trials required for this purpose should be carried out under conditions affording the best possible protection for the subjects. Criteria for the protection of children in clinical trials therefore need to be laid down.

(4) In the case of other persons incapable of giving their consent, such as persons with dementia, psychiatric patients, etc., inclusion in clinical trials in such cases should be on an even more restrictive basis. Medicinal products for trial may be administered to all such individuals only when there are grounds for

[1] OJ L 147, 9.6.1975, p.1. Directive as last amended by Commission Directive 1999/83/EC (OJ L 243, 15.9.1999, p.9).

assuming that the direct benefit to the patient outweighs the risks. Moreover, in such cases the written consent of the patient's legal representative, given in cooperation with the treating doctor, is necessary before participation in any such clinical trial.

(5) The notion of legal representative refers back to existing national law and consequently may include natural or legal persons, an authority and/or a body provided for by national law.

(6) In order to achieve optimum protection of health, obsolete or repetitive tests will not be carried out, whether within the Community or in third countries. The harmonisation of technical requirements for the development of medicinal products should therefore be pursued through the appropriate fora, in particular the International Conference on Harmonisation.

(7) For medicinal products falling within the scope of Part A of the Annex to Council Regulation (EEC)No 2309/93 of 22 July 1993 laying down Community procedures for the authorisation and supervision of medicinal products for human and veterinary use and establishing a European Agency for the Evaluation of Medicinal Products[1], which include products intended for gene therapy or cell therapy, prior scientific evaluation by the European Agency for the Evaluation of Medicinal Products (hereinafter referred to as the 'Agency'), assisted by the Committee for Proprietary Medicinal Products, is mandatory before the Commission grants marketing authorisation. In the course of this evaluation, the said Committee may request full details of the results of the clinical trials on which the application for marketing authorisation is based and, consequently, on the manner in which these trials were conducted and the same Committee may go so far as to require the applicant for such authorisation to conduct further clinical trials. Provision must therefore be made to allow the Agency to have full information on the conduct of any clinical trial for such medicinal products.

(8) A single opinion for each Member State concerned reduces delay in the commencement of a trial without jeopardising the well-being of the people participating in the trial or excluding the possibility of rejecting it in specific sites.

(9) Information on the content, commencement and termination of a

---

[1] OJ L 214, 24.8.1993, p.1. Regulation as amended by Commission Regulation (EC)No 649/98 (OJ L 88, 24.3.1998, p.7)

clinical trial should be available to the Member States where the trial takes place and all the other Member States should have access to the same information. A European database bringing together this information should therefore be set up, with due regard for the rules of confidentiality.

(10) Clinical trials are a complex operation, generally lasting one or more years, usually involving numerous participants and several trial sites, often in different Member States. Member States' current practices diverge considerably on the rules on commencement and conduct of the clinical trials and the requirements for carrying them out vary widely. This therefore results in delays and complications detrimental to effective conduct of such trials in the Community. It is therefore necessary to simplify and harmonise the administrative provisions governing such trials by establishing a clear, transparent procedure and creating conditions conducive to effective coordination of such clinical trials in the Community by the authorities concerned.

(11) As a rule, authorisation should be implicit, i.e. if there has been a vote in favour by the Ethics Committee and the competent authority has not objected within a given period, it should be possible to begin the clinical trials. In excep-tional cases raising especially complex problems, explicit written authorisation should, however, be required.

(12) The principles of good manufacturing practice should be applied to investigational medicinal products.

(13) Special provisions should be laid down for the labelling of these products.

(14) Non-commercial clinical trials conducted by researchers without the participation of the pharmaceuticals industry may be of great benefit to the patients concerned. The Directive should therefore take account of the special position of trials whose planning does not require particular manufacturing or packaging processes, if these trials are carried out with medicinal products with a marketing authorisation within the meaning of Directive 65/65/EEC, manufactured or import-ed in accordance with the provisions of Directives 75/319/EEC and 91/356/EEC, and on patients with the same characteristics as those covered by the indication specified in this marketing authorisation. Labelling of the investigational medicinal products intended for trials of this nature should be subject to simplified provisions laid down in the good manufacturing practice guidelines on investigational products and in Directive 91/ 356/EEC.

(15) The verification of compliance with the standards of good clinical practice and the need to subject data, information and documents to inspection in order to confirm that they have been properly generated, recorded and reported are essential in order to justify the involvement of human subjects in clinical trials.

(16) The person participating in a trial must consent to the scrutiny of personal information during inspection by competent authorities and properly authorised persons, provided that such personal information is treated as strictly confidential and is not made publicly available.

(17) This Directive is to apply without prejudice to Directive 95/46/EEC of the European Parliament and of the Council of 24 October 1995 on the protection of individuals with regard to the processing of personal data and on the free movement of such data[1].

(18) It is also necessary to make provision for the monitoring of adverse reactions occurring in clinical trials using Community surveillance (pharmacovigilance) procedures in order to ensure the immediate cessation of any clinical trial in which there is an unacceptable level of risk.

(19) The measures necessary for the implementation of this Directive should be adopted in accordance with Council Decision 1999/468/EC of 28 June 1999 laying down the procedures for the exercise of implementing powers conferred on the Commission[2],

HAVE ADOPTED THIS DIRECTIVE:

Article 1

Scope

1. This Directive establishes specific provisions regarding the conduct of clinical trials, including multi-centre trials, on human subjects involving medicinal products as defined in Article 1 of Directive 65/65/EEC, in particular relating to the implementation of good clinical practice. This Directive does not apply to non-interventional trials.

2. Good clinical practice is a set of internationally recognised ethical and scientific quality requirements which must be observed for designing, conducting, recording and reporting clinical trials that involve the participation of human subjects. Compliance with this good practice provides assurance that the rights, safety and well-being of trial subjects

[1] OJ L 281, 23.11.1995, p.31.
[2] OJ L 184, 17.7.1999, p.23.

are protected, and that the results of the clinical trials are credible.

3. The principles of good clinical practice and detailed guidelines in line with those principles shall be adopted and, if necessary, revised to take account of technical and scientific progress in accordance with the procedure referred to in Article 21(2).

These detailed guidelines shall be published by the Commission.

4. All clinical trials, including bioavailability and bioequivalence studies, shall be designed, conducted and reported in accordance with the principles of good clinical practice.

Article 2

Definitions

For the purposes of this Directive the following definitions shall apply:

(a) 'clinical trial': any investigation in human subjects intended to discover or verify the clinical, pharmacological and/or other pharmacodynamic effects of one or more investigational medicinal product(s), and/or to identify any adverse reactions to one or more investigational medicinal product(s) and/or to study absorption, distribution, metabolism and excretion of one or more investigational medicinal product(s) with the object of ascertaining its (their) safety and/or efficacy;

This includes clinical trials carried out in either one site or multiple sites, whether in one or more than one Member State;

(b) 'multi-centre clinical trial': a clinical trial conducted according to a single protocol but at more than one site, and therefore by more than one investigator, in which the trial sites may be located in a single Member State, in a number of Member States and/or in Member States and third countries;

(c) 'non-interventional trial': a study where the medicinal product(s) is (are) prescribed in the usual manner in accordance with the terms of the marketing authorisation. The assignment of the patient to a particular therapeutic strategy is not decided in advance by a trial protocol but falls within current practice and the prescription of the medicine is clearly separated from the decision to include the patient in the study. No additional diagnostic or monitoring procedures shall be applied to the patients and epidemiological methods shall be used for the analysis of collected data;

(d) 'investigational medicinal product': a pharmaceutical form of an active substance or placebo being tested or used as a reference in a clinical trial, including products already with a marketing authorisation but used or assembled (formulated or packaged) in a way different from the authorised form, or when used for an unauthorised indication, or when used to gain further information about the authorised form;

(e) 'sponsor': an individual, company, institution or organisation which takes responsibility for the initiation, management and/or financing of a clinical trial;

(f) 'investigator': a doctor or a person following a profession agreed in the Member State for investigations because of the scientific background and the experience in patient care it requires. The investigator is responsible for the conduct of a clinical trial at a trial site. If a trial is conducted by a team of individuals at a trial site, the investigator is the leader responsible for the team and may be called the principal investigator;

(g) 'investigator's brochure': a compilation of the clinical and non-clinical data on the investigational medicinal product or products which are relevant to the study of the product or products in human subjects;

(h) 'protocol': a document that describes the objective(s), design, methodology, statistical considerations and organisation of a trial. The term protocol refers to the protocol, successive versions of the protocol and protocol amendments;

(i) 'subject': an individual who participates in a clinical trial as either a recipient of the investigational medicinal product or a control;

(j) 'informed consent': decision, which must be written, dated and signed, to take part in a clinical trial, taken freely after being duly informed of its nature, significance, implications and risks and appropriately documented, by any person capable of giving consent or, where the person is not capable of giving consent, by his or her legal representative; if the person concerned is unable to write, oral consent in the presence of at least one witness may be given in exceptional cases, as provided for in national legislation.

(k) 'ethics committee': an independent body in a Member State, consisting of healthcare professionals and non-medical members, whose responsibility it is to protect the rights, safety and well-being of human subjects involved in a trial and to provide public assurance of that protection, by, among other things, expressing an opinion on the trial protocol, the suitability of the investigators and the adequacy of facilities, and on the methods and documents to be used to inform trial subjects and obtain their informed consent;

(l) 'inspection': the act by a competent authority of conducting an official review of documents, facilities, records, quality assurance arrangements, and any other resources that are deemed by the competent authority to be related to the clinical trial and that may be located at the site of the trial, at the sponsor's and/or contract research organisation's facilities, or at other establishments which the competent authority sees fit to inspect;

(m) 'adverse event': any untoward medical occurrence in a patient or clinical trial subject administered a medicinal product and which does not necessarily have a causal relationship with this treatment;

(n) 'adverse reaction': all untoward and unintended responses to an investigational medicinal product related to any dose administered;

(o) 'serious adverse event or serious adverse reaction': any untoward medical occurrence or effect that at any dose results in death, is life-threatening, requires hospitalisation or prolongation of existing hospitalisa-

tion, results in persistent or significant disability or incapacity, or is a congenital anomaly or birth defect;

(p) 'unexpected adverse reaction': an adverse reaction, the nature or severity of which is not consistent with the applicable product information (e.g. investigator's brochure for an unauthorised investigational product or summary of product characteristics for an authorised product).

Article 3

Protection of clinical trial subjects

1. This Directive shall apply without prejudice to the national provisions on the protection of clinical trial subjects if they are more comprehensive than the provisions of this Directive and consistent with the procedures and time-scales specified therein. Member States shall, insofar as they have not already done so, adopt detailed rules to protect from abuse individuals who are incapable of giving their informed consent.

2. A clinical trial may be undertaken only if, in particular:

(a) the foreseeable risks and inconveniences have been weighed against the anticipated benefit for the individual trial subject and other present and future patients. A clinical trial may be initiated only if the Ethics Committee and/or the competent authority comes to the conclusion that the anticipated therapeutic and public health benefits justify the risks and may be continued only if compliance with this requirement is permanently monitored;

(b) the trial subject or, when the person is not able to give informed consent, his legal representative has had the opportunity, in a prior interview with the investigator or a member of the investigating team, to understand the objectives, risks and inconveniences of the trial, and the conditions under which it is to be conducted and has also been informed of his right to withdraw from the trial at any time;

(c) the rights of the subject to physical and mental integrity, to privacy and to the protection of the data concerning him in accordance with Directive 95/46/EC are safeguarded;

(d) the trial subject or, when the person is not able to give informed consent, his legal representative has given his written consent after being informed of the nature, significance, implications and risks of the clinical trial; if the individual is unable to write, oral consent in the presence of at least one witness may

be given in exceptional cases, as provided for in national legislation;

(e) the subject may without any resulting detriment withdraw from the clinical trial at any time by revoking his informed consent;

(f) provision has been made for insurance or indemnity to cover the liability of the investigator and sponsor.

3. The medical care given to, and medical decisions made on behalf of, subjects shall be the responsibility of an appropriately qualified doctor or, where appropriate, of a qualified dentist.

4. The subject shall be provided with a contact point where he may obtain further information.

Article 4

Clinical trials on minors

In addition to any other relevant restriction, a clinical trial on minors may be undertaken only if:

(a) the informed consent of the parents or legal representative has been obtained; consent must represent the minor's presumed will and may be revoked at any time, without detriment to the minor;

(b) the minor has received information according to its capacity of understanding, from staff with experience with minors, regarding the trial, the risks and the benefits;

(c) the explicit wish of a minor who is capable of forming an opinion and assessing this information to refuse participation or to be withdrawn from the clinical trial at any time is considered by the investigator or where appropriate the principal investigator;

(d) no incentives or financial inducements are given except compensation;

(e) some direct benefit for the group of patients is obtained from the clinical trial and only where such research is essential to validate data obtained in clinical trials on persons able to give informed consent or by other research methods; additionally, such research should either relate directly to a clinical condition from which the minor concerned suffers or be of such a nature that it can only be carried out on minors;

(f) the corresponding scientific guidelines of the Agency have been followed;

(g) clinical trials have been designed to minimise pain, discomfort, fear and any other foreseeable risk in relation to the disease and developmental stage; both the risk threshold and the degree of distress have to be specially defined and constantly monitored;

(h) the Ethics Committee, with paediatric expertise or after taking advice in clinical, ethical and psychosocial problems in the field of paediatrics, has endorsed the protocol; and

(i) the interests of the patient always prevail over those of science and society.

Article 5

Clinical trials on incapacitated adults not able to give informed legal consent

In the case of other persons incapable of giving informed legal consent, all relevant requirements listed for persons capable of giving such consent shall apply. In addition to these requirements, inclusion in clinical trials of incapacitated adults who have not given or not refused informed consent before the onset of their incapacity shall be allowed only if:

(a) the informed consent of the legal representative has been obtained; consent must represent the subject's presumed will and may be revoked at any time, without detriment to the subject;

(b) the person not able to give informed legal consent has

received information according to his/her capacity of understanding regarding the trial, the risks and the benefits;

(c) the explicit wish of a subject who is capable of forming an opinion and assessing this information to refuse participation in, or to be withdrawn from, the clinical trial at any time is considered by the investigator or where appropriate the principal investigator;

(d) no incentives or financial inducements are given except compensation;

(e) such research is essential to validate data obtained in clinical trials on persons able to give informed consent or by other research methods and relates directly to a life-threatening or debilitating clinical condition from which the incapacitated adult concerned suffers;

(f) clinical trials have been designed to minimise pain, discomfort, fear and any other foreseeable risk in relation to the disease and developmental stage; both the risk threshold and the degree of distress shall be specially defined and constantly monitored;

(g) the Ethics Committee, with expertise in the relevant disease and the patient population concerned or after taking advice in clinical, ethical and psychosocial questions in the field of the relevant disease and patient population concerned, has endorsed the protocol;

(h) the interests of the patient always prevail over those of science and society; and

(i) there are grounds for expecting that administering the medicinal product to be tested will produce a benefit to the patient outweighing the risks or produce no risk at all.

Article 6

Ethics Committee

1. For the purposes of implementation of the clinical trials, Member States shall take the measures necessary for establishment and operation of Ethics Committees.

2. The Ethics Committee shall give its opinion, before a clinical trial commences, on any issue requested.

3. In preparing its opinion, the Ethics Committee shall consider, in particular:

(a) the relevance of the clinical trial and the trial design;

(b) whether the evaluation of the anticipated benefits and risks as required under Article 3(2)(a) is satisfactory and whether the conclusions are justified;

(c) the protocol;

(d) the suitability of the investigator and supporting staff;

(e) the investigator's brochure;

(f) the quality of the facilities;

(g) the adequacy and completeness of the written information to be given and the procedure to be followed for the purpose of obtaining informed consent and the justification for the research on persons incapable of giving informed consent as regards the specific restrictions laid down in Article 3;

(h) provision for indemnity or compensation in the event of injury or death attributable to a clinical trial;

(i) any insurance or indemnity to cover the liability of the investigator and sponsor;

(j) the amounts and, where appropriate, the arrangements for rewarding or compensating investigators and trial subjects and the relevant aspects of any agreement between the sponsor and the site;

(k) the arrangements for the recruitment of subjects.

4. Notwithstanding the provisions of this Article, a Member State may decide that the competent authority it has designated for the purpose of Article 9 shall be responsible for the consideration of, and the giving of an opinion on, the matters referred to in paragraph 3(h), (i) and (j) of this Article.

When a Member State avails itself of this provision, it shall notify the Commission, the other Member States and the Agency.

5. The Ethics Committee shall have a maximum of 60 days from the date of receipt of a valid application to give its reasoned opinion to the applicant and the competent authority in the Member State concerned.

6. Within the period of examination of the application for an opinion, the Ethics Committee may send a single request for information supplementary to that already supplied by the applicant. The period laid down in paragraph 5 shall be suspended until receipt of the supplementary information.

7. No extension to the 60-day period referred to in paragraph 5 shall be permissible except in the case of trials involving medicinal products for gene therapy or somatic cell therapy or medicinal products containing genetically modified organisms. In this case, an extension of a maximum of 30 days shall be permitted. For these products, this 90-day period may be extended by a further 90 days in the event of consultation of a group or a committee in accordance with the regulations and procedures of the Member States concerned. In the case of xenogenic cell therapy, there shall be

no time limit to the authorisation period.

Article 7

Single opinion

For multi-centre clinical trials limited to the territory of a single Member State, Member States shall establish a procedure providing, notwithstanding the number of Ethics Committees, for the adoption of a single opinion for that Member State. In the case of multi-centre clinical trials carried out in more than one Member State simultaneously, a single opinion shall be given for each Member State concerned by the clinical trial.

Article 8

Detailed guidance

The Commission, in consultation with Member States and interested parties, shall draw up and publish detailed guidance on the application format and documentation to be submitted in an application for an ethics committee opinion, in particular regarding the information that is given to subjects, and on the appropriate safeguards for the protection of personal data.

Article 9

Commencement of a clinical trial

1. Member States shall take the measures necessary to ensure that the procedure described in this Article is followed for commencement of a clinical trial. The sponsor may not start a clinical trial until the Ethics Committee has issued a favourable opinion and inasmuch as the competent authority of the Member State concerned has not informed the sponsor of any grounds for non-acceptance. The procedures to reach these decisions can be run in parallel or not, depending on the sponsor.

2. Before commencing any clinical trial, the sponsor shall be required to submit a valid request for authorisation to the competent authority of the Member State in which the sponsor plans to conduct the clinical trial.

3. If the competent authority of the Member State notifies the sponsor of grounds for non-acceptance, the sponsor may, on one occasion only, amend the content of the request referred to in paragraph 2 in order to take due account of the grounds given. If the sponsor fails to amend the request accordingly, the request shall be considered rejected and the clinical trial may not commence.

4. Consideration of a valid request for authorisation by the competent authority as stated in paragraph 2 shall be carried out as rapidly as possible and may not exceed 60 days. The Member States may lay down a shorter period than 60 days within their area of responsibility if that is in compliance with current practice. The competent authority can nevertheless notify the sponsor before the end of this period that it has no grounds for non-acceptance.

No further extensions to the period referred to in the first subparagraph shall be permissible except in the case of trials involving the medicinal products listed in paragraph 6, for which an extension of a maximum of 30 days shall be permitted. For these products, this 90-day period may be extended by a further 90 days in the event of consultation of a group or a committee in accordance with the regulations and procedures of the Member States concerned. In the case of xenogenic cell therapy there shall be no time limit to the authorisation period.

5. Without prejudice to paragraph 6, written authorisation may be required before the commencement of clinical trials for such trials on medicinal products which do not have a marketing authorisation with-in the meaning of Directive 65/65/EEC and are referred to in Part A of the Annex to Regulation (EEC)No 2309/93, and other medicinal products with special characteristics, such as medicinal products the active ingredient or active ingredients of which is or are a biological product or biological products of human or animal origin, or contains biological components of human or animal origin, or the manufacturing of which requires such components.

6. Written authorisation shall be required before commencing clinical trials involving medicinal products for gene therapy, somatic cell therapy including xenogenic cell therapy and all medicinal products containing genetically modified organisms. No gene therapy trials may be carried out which result in modifications to the subject's germ line genetic identity.

7. This authorisation shall be issued without prejudice to the application of Council Directives 90/219/EEC of 23 April 1990 on the contained use of genetically modified micro-organisms[1] and 90/220/EEC of 23 April 1990 on the deliberate release into the environment of genetically modified organisms[1].

8. In consultation with Member States, the Commission shall draw

---

[1] OJ L 117, 8. 5. 1990, p.1. Directive as last amended by Directive 98/81/EC (OJ L 330, 5.12.1998, p.13).

up and publish detailed guidance on:

(a) the format and contents of the request referred to in paragraph 2 as well as the documentation to be submitted to support that request, on the quality and manufacture of the investigational medicinal product, any toxicological and pharmacological tests, the protocol and clinical information on the investigational medicinal product including the investigator's brochure;

(b) the presentation and content of the proposed amendment referred to in point (a) of Article 10 on substantial amendments made to the protocol;

(c) the declaration of the end of the clinical trial.

Article 10

Conduct of a clinical trial

Amendments may be made to the conduct of a clinical trial following the procedure described hereinafter:

(a) after the commencement of the clinical trial, the sponsor may make amendments to the protocol. If those amendments are substantial and are likely to have an impact on the safety of the trial subjects or to change the interpretation of the scientific documents in support of the conduct of the trial, or if they are otherwise significant, the sponsor shall notify the competent authorities of the Member State or Member States concerned of the reasons for, and content of, these amendments and shall inform the ethics committee or committees concerned in accordance with Articles 6 and 9.

On the basis of the details referred to in Article 6(3) and in accordance with Article 7, the Ethics Committee shall give an opinion within a maximum of 35 days of the date of receipt of the proposed amendment in good and due form. If this opinion is unfavourable, the sponsor may not implement the amendment to the protocol.

If the opinion of the Ethics Committee is favourable and the competent authorities of the Member States have raised no grounds for non-acceptance of the above mentioned substantial amendments, the sponsor shall proceed to conduct the clinical trial following the amended protocol. Should this not be the

---

[1] OJ L 117, 8. 5. 1990, p.15. Directive as last amended by Commission Directive 97/35/EC (OJ L 169, 27.6.1997, p. 72).

case, the sponsor shall either take account of the grounds for non-acceptance and adapt the proposed amendment to the protocol accordingly or withdraw the proposed amendment;

(b) without prejudice to point (a), in the light of the circumstances, notably the occurrence of any new event relating to the conduct of the trial or the development of the investigational medicinal product where that new event is likely to affect the safety of the subjects, the sponsor and the investigator shall take appropriate urgent safety measures to protect the subjects against any immediate hazard. The sponsor shall forthwith inform the competent authorities of those new events and the measures taken and shall ensure that the Ethics Committee is notified at the same time;

(c) within 90 days of the end of a clinical trial the sponsor shall notify the competent authorities of the Member State or Member States concerned and the Ethics Committee that the clinical trial has ended. If the trial has to be terminated early, this period shall be reduced to 15 days and the reasons clearly explained.

Article 11

Exchange of information

1. Member States in whose territory the clinical trial takes place shall enter in a European database, accessible only to the competent authorities of the Member States, the Agency and the Commission:

(a) extracts from the request for authorisation referred to in Article 9(2);

(b) any amendments made to the request, as provided for in Article 9(3);

(c) any amendments made to the protocol, as provided for in point a of Article 10;

(d) the favourable opinion of the Ethics Committee;

(e) the declaration of the end of the clinical trial; and

(f) a reference to the inspections carried out on conformity with good clinical practice.

2. At the substantiated request of any Member State, the Agency or the Commission, the competent authority to which the request for authorisation was submitted shall supply all further information concerning the clinical trial in question other than the data already in the European database.

3. In consultation with the Member States, the Commission shall draw

up and publish detailed guidance on the relevant data to be included in this European database, which it operates with the assistance of the Agency, as well as the methods for electronic communication of the data. The detailed guidance thus drawn up shall ensure that the confidentiality of the data is strictly observed.

Article 12

Suspension of the trial or infringements

1. Where a Member State has objective grounds for considering that the conditions in the request for authorisation referred to in Article 9(2) are no longer met or has information raising doubts about the safety or scientific validity of the clinical trial, it may suspend or prohibit the clinical trial and shall notify the sponsor thereof.

Before the Member State reaches its decision it shall, except where there is imminent risk, ask the sponsor and/or the investigator for their opinion, to be delivered within one week.

In this case, the competent authority concerned shall forthwith inform the other competent authorities, the Ethics Committee concerned, the Agency and the Commission of its decision to suspend or prohibit the trial and of the reasons for the decision.

2. Where a competent authority has objective grounds for considering that the sponsor or the investigator or any other person involved in the conduct of the trial no longer meets the obligations laid down, it shall forthwith inform him thereof, indicating the course of action which he must take to remedy this state of affairs. The competent authority concerned shall forthwith inform the Ethics Committee, the other competent authorities and the Commission of this course of action.

Article 13

Manufacture and import of investigational medicinal products

1. Member States shall take all appropriate measures to ensure that the manufacture or importation of investigational medicinal products is subject to the holding of authorisation. In order to obtain the authorisation, the applicant and, subsequently, the holder of the authorisation, shall meet at least the requirements defined in accordance with the procedure referred to in Article 21(2).

2. Member States shall take all appropriate measures to ensure that

the holder of the authorisation referred to in paragraph 1 has permanently and continuously at his disposal the services of at least one qualified person who, in accordance with the conditions laid down in Article 23 of the second Council Directive 75/319/EEC of 20 May 1975 on the approximation of provisions laid down by law, regulation or administrative action relating to proprietary medicinal products[1], is responsible in particular for carrying out the duties specified in paragraph 3 of this Article.

3. Member States shall take all appropriate measures to ensure that the qualified person referred to in Article 21 of Directive 75/319/EEC, without prejudice to his relationship with the manufacturer or importer, is responsible, in the context of the procedures referred to in Article 25 of the said Directive, for ensuring:

(a) in the case of investigational medicinal products manufactured in the Member State concerned, that each batch of medicinal products has been manufactured and checked in compliance with the requirements of Commission Directive 91/356/EEC of 13 June 1991 laying down the principles and guidelines of good manufacturing practice for medicinal products for human use[2], the product specification file and the information notified pursuant to Article 9(2) of this Directive;

(b) in the case of investigational medicinal products manufactured in a third country, that each production batch has been manufactured and checked in accordance with standards of good manufacturing practice at least equivalent to those laid down in Commission Directive 91/356/EEC, in accordance with the product specification file, and that each production batch has been checked in accordance with the information notified pursuant to Article 9(2) of this Directive;

(c) in the case of an investigational medicinal product which is a comparator product from a third country, and which has a marketing authorisation, where the documentation certifying that each production batch has been manufactured in conditions at least equivalent to the standards of good manufacturing practice referred to above cannot be obtained, that each production batch has undergone all relevant analyses, tests or checks necessary to confirm its quality

---

[1] OJ L 147, 9. 6. 1975, p. 13. Directive as last amended by Council Directive 93/39/EC (OJ L 214, 24. 8. 1993, p. 22).

[2] OJ L 193, 17. 7. 1991, p. 30.

in accordance with the information notified pursuant to Article 9(2) of this Directive.

Detailed guidance on the elements to be taken into account when evaluating products with the object of releasing batches within the Community shall be drawn up pursuant to the good manufacturing practice guidelines, and in particular Annex 13 to the said guidelines. Such guidelines will be adopted in accordance with the procedure referred to in Article 21(2) of this Directive and published in accordance with Article 19a of Directive 75/319/EEC.

Insofar as the provisions laid down in (a), (b) or (c) are complied with, investigational medicinal products shall not have to undergo any further checks if they are imported into another Member State together with batch release certification signed by the qualified person.

4. In all cases, the qualified person must certify in a register or equivalent document that each production batch satisfies the provisions of this Article. The said register or equivalent document shall be kept up to date as operations are carried out and shall remain at the disposal of the agents of the competent authority for the period specified in the provisions of the Member States concerned. This period shall in any event be not less than five years.

5. Any person engaging in activities as the qualified person referred to in Article 21 of Directive 75/319/EEC as regards investigational medicinal products at the time when this Directive is applied in the Member State where that person is, but without complying with the conditions laid down in Articles 23 and 24 of that Directive, shall be authorised to continue those activities in the Member State concerned.

Article 14

Labelling

The particulars to appear in at least the official language(s) of the Member State on the outer packaging of investigational medicinal products or, where there is no outer packaging, on the immediate packaging, shall be published by the Commission in the good manufacturing practice guidelines on investigational medicinal products adopted in accordance with Article 19a of Directive 75/319/EEC.

In addition, these guidelines shall lay down adapted provisions relating to labelling for investigational medicinal products intended for clinical trials with the following characteristics:
- the planning of the trial does not require particular manufacturing or packaging processes;

- the trial is conducted with medicinal products with, in the Member States concerned by the study, a marketing authorisation within the meaning of Directive 65/65/EEC, manufactured or imported in accordance with the provisions of Directive 75/319/EEC;

- the patients participating in the trial have the same characteristics as those covered by the indication specified in the above mentioned authorisation.

Article 15

Verification of compliance of investigational medicinal products with good clinical and manufacturing practice

1. To verify compliance with the provisions on good clinical and manufacturing practice, Member States shall appoint inspectors to inspect the sites concerned by any clinical trial conducted, particularly the trial site or sites, the manufacturing site of the investigational medicinal product, any laboratory used for analyses in the clinical trial and/or the sponsor's premises.

The inspections shall be conducted by the competent authority of the Member State concerned, which shall inform the Agency; they shall be carried out on behalf of the Community and the results shall be recognised by all the other Member States. These inspections shall be coordinated by the Agency, within the framework of its powers as provided for in Regulation (EEC)No 2309/93. A Member State may request assistance from another Member State in this matter.

2. Following inspection, an inspection report shall be prepared. It must be made available to the sponsor while safeguarding confidential aspects. It may be made available to the other Member States, to the Ethics Committee and to the Agency, at their reasoned request.

3. At the request of the Agency, within the framework of its powers as provided for in Regulation (EEC)No 2309/93, or of one of the Member States concerned, and following consultation with the Member States concerned, the Commission may request a new inspection should verification of compliance with this Directive reveal differences between Member States.

4. Subject to any arrangements which may have been concluded between the Community and third countries, the Commission, upon receipt of a reasoned request from a Member State or on its own initiative, or a Member State may propose that the trial site and/or the

sponsor's premises and/or the manufacturer established in a third country undergo an inspection. The inspection shall be carried out by duly qualified Community inspectors.

5.   The detailed guidelines on the documentation relating to the clinical trial, which shall constitute the master file on the trial, archiving, qualifications of inspectors and inspection procedures to verify compliance of the clinical trial in question with this Directive shall be adopted and revised in accordance with the procedure referred to in Article 21(2).

requirements and within the time periods specified in the protocol.

3.   For reported deaths of a subject, the investigator shall supply the sponsor and the Ethics Committee with any additional information requested.

4.   The sponsor shall keep detailed records of all adverse events which are reported to him by the investigator or investigators. These records shall be submitted to the Member States in whose territory the clinical trial is being conducted, if they so request.

Article 16

Notification of adverse events

1.   The investigator shall report all serious adverse events immediately to the sponsor except for those that the protocol or investigator's brochure identifies as not requiring immediate reporting. The immediate report shall be followed by detailed, written reports. The immediate and follow-up reports shall identify subjects by unique code numbers assigned to the latter.

2.   Adverse events and/or laboratory abnormalities identified in the protocol as critical to safety evaluations shall be reported to the sponsor according to the reporting

Article 17

Notification of serious adverse reactions

1.(a) The sponsor shall ensure that all relevant information about suspected serious unexpected adverse reactions that are fatal or life-threatening is recorded and reported as soon as possible to the competent authorities in all the Member States concerned, and to the Ethics Committee, and in any case no later than seven days after knowledge by the sponsor of such a case, and that relevant follow-up information is subsequently communicated within an additional eight days.

(b) All other suspected serious unexpected adverse reactions shall be reported to the competent authorities concerned and to the Ethics Committee concerned as soon as possible but within a maximum of fifteen days of first knowledge by the sponsor.

(c) Each Member State shall ensure that all suspected unexpected serious adverse reactions to an investigational medicinal product which are brought to its attention are recorded.

(d) The sponsor shall also inform all investigators.

2. Once a year throughout the clinical trial, the sponsor shall provide the Member States in whose territory the clinical trial is being conducted and the Ethics Committee with a listing of all suspected serious adverse reactions which have occurred over this period and a report of the subjects safety.

3.(a) Each Member State shall see to it that all suspected unexpected serious adverse reactions to an investigational medicinal product which are brought to its attention are immediately entered in a European database to which, in accordance with Article 11(1), only the competent authorities of the Member States, the Agency and the Commission shall have access.

(b) The Agency shall make the information notified by the sponsor available to the competent authorities of the Member States.

Article 18

Guidance concerning reports

The Commission, in consultation with the Agency, Member States and interested parties, shall draw up and publish detailed guidance on the collection, verification and presentation of adverse event/reaction reports, together with decoding procedures for unexpected serious adverse reactions.

Article 19

General provisions

This Directive is without prejudice to the civil and criminal liability of the sponsor or the investigator. To this end, the sponsor or a legal representative of the sponsor must be established in the Community.

Unless Member States have established precise conditions for exceptional circumstances, investigational medicinal products and, as the case may be, the devices used for their administration shall be made available free of charge by the sponsor.

The Member States shall inform the Commission of such conditions.

Article 20

Adaptation to scientific and technical progress

This Directive shall be adapted to take account of scientific and technical progress in accordance with the procedure referred to in Article 21(2).

Article 21

Committee procedure

1. The Commission shall be assisted by the Standing Committee on Medicinal Products for Human Use, set up by Article 2b of Directive 75/318/EEC (hereinafter referred to as the Committee).

2. Where reference is made to this paragraph, Articles 5 and 7 of Decision 1999/468/EC shall apply, having regard to the provisions of Article 8 thereof.

The period referred to in Article 5(6) of Decision 1999/468/EC shall be set at three months.

3. The Committee shall adopt its rules of procedure.

Article 22

Application

1. Member States shall adopt and publish before 1 May 2003 the laws, regulations and administrative provisions necessary to comply with this Directive. They shall forthwith inform the Commission thereof.

They shall apply these provisions at the latest with effect from 1 May 2004.

When Member States adopt these provisions, they shall contain a reference to this Directive or shall be accompanied by such reference on the occasion of their official publication. The methods of making such reference shall be laid down by Member States.

2. Member States shall communicate to the Commission the text of the provisions of national law which they adopt in the field governed by this Directive.

Article 23

Entry into force

This Directive shall enter into force on the day of its publication in the Official Journal of the European Communities.

Article 24

Addressees

This Directive is addressed to the
Member States.

Done at Luxembourg, 4 April 2001.

For the European Parliament –
The President – N. FONTAINE
For the Council – The President –
B. ROSENGREN

COMMISSION DIRECTIVE 2005/28/EC of 8 April 2005

laying down principles and detailed guidelines for good clinical practice as regards investigational medicinal products for human use, as well as the requirements for authorisation of the manufacturing or importation of such products

THE COMMISSION OF THE EUROPEAN COMMUNITIES,

Having regard to the Treaty establishing the European Community,

Having regard to Directive 2001/20/EC of the European Parliament and of the Council of 4 April 2001 on the approximation of the laws, regulations and administrative provisions of the Member States relating to the implementation of good clinical practice in the conduct of clinical trials on medicinal products for human use[1], and in particular Article 1(3), Article 13(1) and Article 15(5) thereof, Whereas:

(1) Directive 2001/20/EC requires the adoption of principles of good clinical practice and detailed guidelines in line with those principles, minimum requirements for authorisation of the manufacture or importation of investigational medicinal products, and detailed guidelines on the documentation relating to clinical trials to verify their compliance with Directive 2001/20/EC.

(2) The principles and guidelines for good clinical practice should be such as to ensure that the conduct of clinical trials on investigational medicinal products, as defined in Article 2(d) of Directive 2001/20/EC, is founded in the protection of human rights and the dignity of the human being.

(3) Manufacturing requirements to be applied to investigational medicinal products are provided for by Commission Directive 2003/94/EC of 8 October 2003 laying down the principles and guidelines of good manufacturing practice in respect of medicinal products for human use and investigational medicinal products for human use[2]. Title IV of Directive 2001/83/EC of the European Parliament and of

---

[1] OJ L 121, 1.5.2001, p. 34.
[2] OJ L 262, 14.10.2003, p. 22.

the Council of 6 November 2001 on the Community code relating to medicinal products for human use[1] contains the provisions applied for the authorisation for the manufacture of medicinal products as part of the requirements needed for the application for a marketing authorisation. Article 3 (3) of that Directive establishes that these requirements are not applicable for medicinal products intended for research and development trials. It is therefore necessary to lay down minimal requirements regarding applications for and management of authorisations to manufacture or import investigational medicinal products, as well as for the granting and the content of the authorisations, in order to guarantee the quality of the investigational medicinal product used in the clinical trial.

(4) With regard to the protection of trial subjects and to ensure that unnecessary clinical trials will not be conducted, it is important to define principles and detailed guidelines of good clinical practice whilst allowing the results of the trials to be documented for use in a later phase.

(5) To ensure that all experts and individuals involved in the design, initiation, conduct and recording of clinical trials apply the same standards of good clinical practice, principles and detailed guidelines of good clinical practice have to be defined.

(6) Provisions for the functioning of the Ethics Committees should be established in each Member State on the basis of common detailed guidelines, in order to ensure the protection of the trial subject while at the same time allowing a harmonised application in the different Member States of the procedures to be used by Ethics Committees.

(7) To secure the compliance of clinical trials with the provisions on good clinical practice, it is necessary that inspectors ensure the practical effectiveness of such provisions. It is essential therefore to provide detailed guidelines on the minimum standards for the qualification of inspectors, in particular as regards their education and training. For the same reason, detailed guidelines on inspection procedures, in particular on the cooperation of the various agencies, and the follow-up to the inspections, should be laid down.

(8) The International Conference on Harmonisation (ICH) reached a consensus in 1995 to provide a har-

---

[1] OJ L 311, 28.11.2003, p. 67. Directive as last amended by Directive 2004/27/EC (OJ L 136, 30.4.2004, p. 34).

monised approach for Good Clinical Practice. The consensus paper should be taken into account as agreed upon by the Committee for Medicinal Products for Human Use (CHMP) of the European Medicines Agency, hereinafter 'the Agency', and published by the Agency.

(9) It is necessary that sponsors, investigators and other participants take into account the scientific guidelines relating to the quality, safety and efficacy of medicinal products for human use, as agreed upon by the CHMP and published by the Agency, as well as the other pharmaceutical Community guidelines published by the Commission in the different volumes of The rules governing medicinal products in the European Community.

(10) In conducting clinical trials on investigational medicinal products for human use, the safety and the protection of the rights of trial subjects should be ensured. The detailed rules adopted by Member States pursuant to Article 3(1) of Directive 2001/20/EC, to protect from abuse individuals who are incapable of giving their informed consent should also cover individuals temporarily incapable of giving their informed consent, as in emergency situations.

(11) Non-commercial clinical trials conducted by researchers without the participation of the pharmaceutical industry may be of great benefit to the patients concerned. Directive 2001/20/EC recognises the specificity of these non-commercial clinical trials. In particular, when trials are conducted with authorised medicinal products and on patients with the same characteristics as those covered by the authorised indication, requirements already fulfilled by these authorised medicinal products, as far as manufacturing or importation are concerned, should be taken into consideration. However, it could also be necessary, due to the specific conditions under which non-commercial trials are conducted, that Member States foresee specific modalities to be applied to these trials not only when conducted with authorised medicinal products and on patients with the same characteristics, in order to comply with the principles imposed by this Directive, in particular as far as the manufacturing or import requirements for authorisation and the documentation to be submitted and archived for the trial master file are concerned.

The conditions under which the noncommercial research is conducted by public researchers and the places where this research takes place, make the application of certain of the details of good clinical practice unnecessary or guaranteed by other means. Member States will ensure in these cases, when providing for specific modalities, that the objectives of the protection of the rights of patients who participate in the trial, as well as, in general, the correct application of the good clinical practice principles, are achieved. The Commission will prepare a draft with guidance in this respect.

(12) The measures provided for in this Directive are in accordance with the opinion of the Standing Committee on Medicinal Products for Human Use,

HAS ADOPTED THIS DIRECTIVE:

Article I

Subject-matter

1. This Directive lays down the following provisions to be applied to investigational medicinal products for human use:

(a) the principles of good clinical practice and detailed guidelines in line with those principles, as referred to in Article 1(3) of Directive 2001/20/EC, for the design, conduct and reporting of clinical trials on human subjects involving such products;

(b) the requirements for authorisation of the manufacture or importation of such products, as provided for in Article 13(1) of Directive 2001/20/EC;

(c) the detailed guidelines, provided for in Article 15(5) of Directive

2001/20/EC, on the documentation relating to clinical trials, archiving, qualifications of inspectors and inspection procedures.

2. When applying the principles, detailed guidelines and requirements referred to in paragraph 1, Member States shall take into account the technical implementing modalities provided for in the detailed guidance published by the Commission in The Rules governing medicinal products in the European Union.

3. When applying the principles, detailed guidelines and requirements referred to in paragraph 1 to non-commercial clinical trials conducted by researchers without the participation of the pharmaceutical industry, Member States may introduce specific modalities in order to take into account the specificity of these trials as far as Chapters 3 and 4 are concerned.

4. Member States may take into account the special position of trials whose planning does not require particular manufacturing or packaging processes, carried out with medicinal products with marketing authorisations within the meaning of Directive 2001/83/EC, manufactured or imported in accordance with the same Directive and conducted on patients with the same characteristics as those covered by the indication specified in the marketing authorisation. Labelling of investigational

medicinal products intended for trials of that nature may be subject to simplified provisions laid down in the good manufacturing practice guidelines on investigational medicinal products. Member States shall inform the Commission as well as the other Member States of any specific modalities implemented in accordance with this paragraph. These modalities will be published by the Commission.

Article 2

Good clinical practice for the design, conduct, recording and reporting of clinical trials

1. The rights, safety and well being of the trial subjects shall prevail over the interests of science and society.

2. Each individual involved in conducting a trial shall be qualified by education, training, and experience to perform his tasks.

3. Clinical trials shall be scientifically sound and guided by ethical principles in all their aspects.

4. The necessary procedures to secure the quality of every aspect of the trials shall be complied with.

Article 3

The available non-clinical and clinical information on an investigational medicinal product shall be adequate to support the proposed clinical trial. Clinical trials shall be conducted in accordance with the Declaration of Helsinki on Ethical Principles for Medical Research Involving Human Subjects, adopted by the General Assembly of the World Medical Association (1996).

Article 4

The protocol referred to in point (h) of Article 2 of Directive 2001/20/EC shall provide for the definition of inclusion and exclusion of subjects participating in a clinical trial, monitoring and publication policy. The investigator and sponsor shall consider all relevant guidance with respect to commencing and conducting a clinical trial.

Article 5

All clinical trial information shall be recorded, handled, and stored in such a way that it can be accurately reported, interpreted and verified, while the confidentiality of records of the trial subjects remains protected.

Article 6

The ethics committee

1. Each Ethics Committee established under Article 6(1) of Directive 2001/20/EC shall adopt the relevant rules of procedure necessary to implement the requirements set out in that Directive and, in particular, in Articles 6 and 7 thereof.

2. The Ethics Committees shall, in every case, retain the essential documents relating to a clinical trial, as referred to in Article 15(5) of Directive 2001/20/EC, for at least three years after completion of that trial. They shall retain the documents for a longer period, where so required under other applicable requirements.

3. Communication of information between the Ethics Committees and the competent authorities of the Member States shall be ensured through appropriate and efficient systems.

Article 7

The sponsors

1. A sponsor may delegate any or all of his trial-related functions to an individual, a company, an institution or an organisation. However, in such cases, the sponsor shall remain responsible for ensuring that the conduct of the trials and the final data generated by those trials comply with Directive 2001/20/EC as

well as this Directive.

2. The investigator and the sponsor may be the same person.

Article 8

Investigator's brochure

1. The information in the investigator's brochure, referred to in Article 2(g) of Directive 2001/20/EC, shall be presented in a concise, simple, objective, balanced and non-promotional form that enables a clinician or potential investigator to understand it and make an unbiased risk-benefit assessment of the appropriateness of the proposed clinical trial. The first subparagraph shall apply also to any update of the investigator's brochure.

2. If the investigational medicinal product has a marketing authorisation, the Summary of Product Characteristics may be used instead of the investigator's brochure.

3. The investigator's brochure shall be validated and updated by the sponsor at least once a year.

Article 9

Manufacturing or import authorisation

1. Authorisation, as provided for in

Article 13(1) of Directive 2001/20/EC, shall be required for both total and partial manufacture of investigational medicinal products, and for the various processes of dividing up, packaging or presentation. Such authorisation shall be required even if the products manufactured are intended for export. Authorisation shall also be required for imports from third countries into a Member State.

2. Authorisation, as provided for in Article 13(1) of Directive 2001/20/EC, shall not be required for reconstitution prior to use or packaging, where those processes are carried out in hospitals, health centres or clinics, by pharmacists or other persons legally authorised in the Member States to carry out such processes and if the investigational medicinal products are intended to be used exclusively in those institutions.

Article 10

1. In order to obtain the authorisation the applicant must meet at least the following requirements:

(a) specify in his application the types of medicinal products and pharmaceutical forms to be manufactured or imported;
(b) specify in his application the relevant manufacture or import operations;
(c) specify in his application, where

relevant as in the case of viral or non-conventional agents' inactivation, the manufacturing process;
(d) specify in his application the place where the products are to be manufactured or have at his disposal, for their manufacture or importation, suitable and sufficient premises, technical equipment and control facilities complying with the requirements of Directive 2003/94/EC as regards the manufacture, control and storage of the products;
(e) have permanently and continuously at his disposal the services of at least one qualified person as referred to in Article 13(2) of Directive 2001/20/EC.

For the purposes of point (a) of the first subparagraph, 'types of medicinal products' include blood products, immunological products, cell therapy products, gene therapy products, biotechnology products, human or animal extracted products, herbal products, homeopathic products, radiopharmaceutical products and products containing chemical active ingredients.

2. The applicant shall provide with his application documentary evidence that he complies with paragraph 1.

Article 11

1. The competent authority shall issue the authorisation only after verifying the accuracy of the particulars provided by the applicant pursuant to Article 10 by the means of an inquiry carried out by its agents.

2. Member States shall take all appropriate measures to ensure that the procedure for granting an authorisation is completed within 90 days of the day on which the competent authority receives a valid application.

3. The competent authority of the Member State may require from the applicant further information concerning the particulars supplied pursuant to Article 10(1), including in particular information concerning the qualified person at the disposal of the applicant in accordance with point (e) of Article 10(1).

Where the competent authority concerned exercises that right, the application of the time-limits laid down in paragraph 2 shall be suspended until the additional data required have been supplied.

Article 12

1. In order to ensure that the requirements laid down in Article 10 are complied with, authorisation may be made conditional on the carrying out of certain obligations imposed either when authorisation is granted or at a later date.

2. An authorisation shall apply only to the premises specified in the application and to the types of medicinal products and pharmaceutical forms specified in that application pursuant to point (a) of Article 10(1).

Article 13

The holder of the authorisation shall at least comply with the following requirements:

(a) to have at his disposal the services of staff that comply with the legal requirements existing in the Member State concerned both as regards manufacture and controls; EN L 91/16 Official Journal of the European Union 9.4.2005

(b) to dispose of the investigational/authorised medicinal products only in accordance with the legislation of the Member State concerned;

(c) to give prior notice to the competent authority of any changes he may wish to make to any of the particulars supplied pursuant Article 10(1) and, in particular, to inform the competent authority immediately if the qualified person referred to in Article 13(2) of Directive 2001/20/EC is replaced unexpectedly;

(d) to allow agents of the competent authority of the Member State concerned access to his premises at any time;

(e) to enable the qualified person referred to in Article 13(2) of Directive 2001/20/EC to carry out his duties, for example by placing at his disposal all the necessary facilities;

(f) to comply with the principles and guidelines for good manufacturing practice for medicinal products as laid down by Community law.

Detailed guidelines in line with the principles referred to in point (f) of the first paragraph will be published by the Commission and revised where necessary to take account of technical and scientific progress.

Article 14

If the holder of the authorisation requests a change in any of the particulars referred to in points (a) to (e) of Article 10(1), the time taken for the procedure relating to the request shall not exceed 30 days. In exceptional cases, this period of time may be extended to 90 days.

Article 15

The competent authority shall suspend or revoke the authorisation, as a whole or in part, if the holder of the authorisation fails at any time to comply with the relevant requirements.

Article 16

The trial master file and archiving

The documentation referred to Article 15(5) of Directive 2001/20/EC as the trial master file shall consist of essential documents, which enable both the conduct of a clinical trial and the quality of the data produced to be evaluated. Those documents shall show whether the investigator and the sponsor have complied with the principles and guidelines of good clinical practice and with the applicable requirements and, in particular, with Annex I to Directive 2001/83/EC.

The trial master file shall provide the basis for the audit by the sponsor's independent auditor and for the inspection by the competent authority.

The content of the essential documents shall be in accordance with the specificities of each phase of the clinical trial.

The Commission shall publish additional guidance in order to specify the content of these documents.

Article 17

The sponsor and the investigator shall retain the essential documents relating to a clinical trial for at least five years after its completion.

They shall retain the documents for a longer period, where so required by other applicable requirements or by an agreement between the sponsor and the investigator.

Essential documents shall be archived in a way that ensures that they are readily available, upon request, to the competent authorities.

The medical files of trial subjects shall be retained in accordance with national legislation and in accordance with the maximum period of time permitted by the hospital, institution or private practice.

Article 18

Any transfer of ownership of the data or of documents shall be documented. The new owner shall assume responsibility for data reten-

tion and archiving in accordance with Article 17.

Article 19

The sponsor shall appoint individuals within its organisation who are responsible for archives.

Access to archives shall be restricted to the named individuals responsible for the archives.

Article 20

The media used to store essential documents shall be such that those documents remain complete and legible throughout the required period of retention and can be made available to the competent authorities upon request.

Any alteration to records shall be traceable.

Article 21

Inspectors

1. The inspectors, appointed by the Member States pursuant to Article 15(1) of Directive 2001/20/EC, shall be made aware of and maintain confidentiality whenever they gain access to confidential information as a result of good clinical practice

inspections in accordance with applicable Community requirements, national laws or international agreements.

2. Member States shall ensure that inspectors have completed education at university level, or have equivalent experience, in medicine, pharmacy, pharmacology, toxicology or other relevant fields.

3. Member States shall ensure that inspectors receive appropriate training, that their training needs are assessed regularly and that appropriate action is taken to maintain and improve their skills.

Member States shall also ensure that the inspectors have knowledge of the principles and processes that apply to the development of medicinal products and clinical research. Inspectors shall also have knowledge of applicable Community and national legislation and guidelines applicable to the conduct of clinical trials and the granting of marketing authorisations.

The inspectors shall be familiar with the procedures and systems for recording clinical data, and with the organisation and regulation of the healthcare system in the relevant Member States and, where appropriate, in third countries.

4. Member States shall maintain up-to-date records of the qualifications, training and experience of each inspector.

5. Each inspector shall be provided with a document setting out standard operating procedures and giving details of the duties, responsibilities and ongoing training requirements. Those procedures shall be maintained up to date.

6. Inspectors shall be provided with suitable means of identification.

7. Each inspector shall sign a statement declaring any financial or other links to the parties to be inspected. That statement shall be taken into consideration when inspectors are to be assigned to a specific inspection.

Article 22

In order to ensure the presence of skills necessary for specific inspections, Member State may appoint teams of inspectors and experts with appropriate qualifications and experience to fulfil collectively the requirements necessary for conducting the inspection.

Article 23

Inspection procedures

1. Good clinical practice inspections

may take place on any of the following occasions:

(a) before, during or after the conduct of clinical trials;
(b) as part of the verification of applications for marketing authorisation;
(c) as a follow-up to the granting of authorisation.

2. In accordance with Article 15(1) and (2) of Directive 2001/20/EC, inspections may be requested and coordinated by the European Medicines Agency within the scope of Regulation (EC) No 726/2004 of the European Parliament and of the Council[1], especially in connection with clinical trials relating to applications through the procedure established by this Regulation.

3. Inspections shall be conducted in accordance with the inspection guidance documents developed to support the mutual recognition of inspection findings within the Community.

4. Improvement and harmonisation of inspection guidance shall be achieved by the Member States, in collaboration with the Commission and the Agency, through joint inspections, agreed processes and procedures and sharing of experience and training.]

Article 24

Member States shall make publicly available within their territories the documents relating to the adoption of good clinical practice principles. They shall establish the legal and administrative framework within which their good clinical practice inspections operate, with definition of the powers of inspectors for entry into clinical trial sites and access to data. In so doing they shall ensure that, on request and where appropriate, inspectors of the competent authority of the other Member States also have access to the clinical trial sites and data. EN L 91/18 Official Journal of the European Union 9.4.2005 (1) OJ L 136, 30.4.2004, p. 1.

Article 25

Member States shall provide for sufficient resources and shall in particular appoint an adequate number of inspectors to ensure effective verification of compliance with good clinical practice.

Article 26

Member States shall establish the relevant procedures for verification of good clinical practice compliance.

---

[1] OJ L 136, 30.4.2004, p. 1.

The procedures shall include the modalities for examining both the study management procedures and the conditions under which clinical trials are planned, performed, monitored and recorded, as well as follow-up measures.

Article 27

Member States shall establish the relevant procedures for the following:

(a) appointing experts for accompanying inspectors in case of need;

(b) requesting inspections/assistance from other Member States, in line with Article 15(1) of Directive 2001/20/EC and for cooperating in inspections in another Member State;

(c) arranging inspections in third countries.

Article 28

Member States shall maintain records of national and, if applicable, international inspections including the good clinical practice compliance status, and of their follow-up.

Article 29

1. In order to harmonise the conduct of inspections by the competent authorities of the different Member States, guidance documents containing the common provisions on the conduct of those inspections shall be published by the Commission after consultation with the Member States.

2. Member States shall ensure that national inspection procedures are in compliance with the guidance documents referred in paragraph 1.

3. The guidance documents referred to in paragraph 1 may be updated regularly according to scientific and technical development.

Article 30

1. Member States shall lay down all necessary rules to ensure that confidentiality is respected by inspectors and other experts. With regard to personal data, the requirements of Directive 95/46/EC of the European Parliament and of the Council[1] shall be respected.

2. Inspection reports shall be made available by the Member States only to the recipients referred to in Article 15(2) of Directive 2001/20/EC, in accordance with national regulations of the Member States and subject to any arrangements concluded between the Community and third countries.

---

[1] OJ L 281, 23.11.1995, p. 31.

Article 31

Final Provisions

1. Member States shall bring into force the laws, regulations and administrative provisions necessary to comply with this Directive by 29 January 2006 at the latest. They shall forthwith communicate to the Commission the text of those provisions and a correlation table between those provisions and this Directive.

When Member States adopt these provisions, they shall contain a reference to this Directive or be accompanied by such a reference on the occasion of their official publication. Member States shall determine how such reference is to be made.

2. Member States shall communicate to the Commission the text of the main provisions of national law which they adopt in the field covered by this Directive.

Article 32

This Directive shall enter into force on the twentieth day following that of its publication in the Official Journal of the European Union.

Article 33

This Directive is addressed to the Member States.

Done at Brussels, 8 April 2005.

For the Commission
Günter VERHEUGEN
Vice-President